ABSOLUTE BEGINNER'S GUIDE

TO

WITHDRAWN

Coaching Youth Basketball

Tom Hanlon

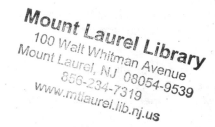
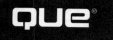

800 East 96th Street,
Indianapolis, Indiana 46240 USA

Absolute Beginner's Guide to Coaching Youth Basketball

International Standard Book Number: 0-7897-3358-7

Library of Congress Catalog Card Number: 2004118410

Printed in the United States of America

First Printing: June 2005

08   07   06   05   4   3   2   1

Trademarks

Warning and Disclaimer

Bulk Sales

Que Publishing offers excellent discounts on this book when ordered in quantity for bulk purchases or special sales. For more information, please contact

U.S. Corporate and Government Sales
1-800-382-3419
corpsales@pearsontechgroup.com

For sales outside the U.S., please contact

International Sales
international@pearsoned.com

Publisher
Paul Boger

Executive Editor
Jeff Riley

Development Editors
Sean Dixon
Steve Rowe

Managing Editor
Charlotte Clapp

Project Editor
Andy Beaster

Production Editor
Heather Wilkins

Indexer
Erika Millen

Proofreader
Lisa Wilson

Technical Editor
Burrall Paye

Publishing Coordinator
Pamalee Nelson

Interior Designer
Anne Jones

Cover Designer
Dan Armstrong

Contents at a Glance

Table of Contents

About the Author

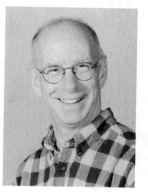

Tom Hanlon has nearly 20 years of professional writing experience as a journalist, editor of two coaching magazines, curriculum writer for a coaching division of a publishing company, and book writer and ghostwriter for nationally-prominent authors. Tom ghostwrote *Teens Can Make It Happen* (Simon & Schuster) for Stedman Graham; this book made the *New York Times* bestseller list in 2000. He has written all or major portions of nearly 40 other books, including seven sport officiating guides and numerous coaches' guides (including baseball, softball, soccer, basketball, and volleyball). Tom has played numerous sports himself and has experience as a youth sport coach. He lives in Champaign, Ill., with his wife, Janet, and children, Tessa and Trevor.

About the Technical Editor

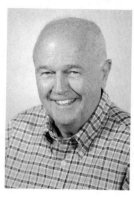

Burrall Paye coached for 37 years and his teams won 65 championships, including a state championship. He earned 42 Coach of the Year awards, including the National Federation Outstanding Coach (1985). Burrall lives with his wife in Roanoke, Virginia.

Dedication

To all the youth basketball coaches who volunteer their time to teach kids the game.

Acknowledgments

Many people used their talents to make this book happen. First and foremost, **Jeff Riley**, executive editor, paved the way for this book, inviting me to write it and getting it approved. I go a long way back with Jeff, though I normally don't admit that in public.

Steve Rowe and **Sean Dixon**, developmental editors, provided consistently excellent advice in shaping the content, in making the book as useful and practical as possible, and in managing all the details and tasks that go into developing a book.

Andy Beaster, project editor and general basketball enthusiast, guided the project through to completion with skill, grace, and élan (read: he kept me on task).

Heather Wilkins lent her considerable talents as a copy editor, cleaning up and tightening the copy.

And **Burrall Paye**, technical editor, provided his expertise throughout the project and created the games and drills in Chapter 11.

We Want to Hear from You!

As the reader of this book, *you* are our most important critic and commentator. We value your opinion and want to know what we're doing right, what we could do better, what areas you'd like to see us publish in, and any other words of wisdom you're willing to pass our way.

As an executive editor for Que Publishing, I welcome your comments. You can email or write me directly to let me know what you did or didn't like about this book—as well as what we can do to make our books better.

Please note that I cannot help you with technical problems related to the topic of this book. We do have a User Services group, however, where I will forward specific technical questions related to the book.

When you write, please be sure to include this book's title and author as well as your name, email address, and phone number. I will carefully review your comments and share them with the author and editors who worked on the book.

Email: feedback@quepublishing.com

Mail: Jeff Riley
              Executive Editor
              Que Publishing
              800 East 96th Street
              Indianapolis, IN 46240 USA

For more information about this book or another Que book, visit our website at www.quepublishing.com. Type the ISBN (excluding hyphens) or the title of a book in the Search field to find the page you're looking for.

INTRODUCTION

It all began so innocently.

Just as the youth basketball league administrator asked for a volunteer to coach your son's team, you scratched the top of your head. All the other parents were studying, with sudden keen interest, their thumbnails or shoelaces. No eyes, except yours, were looking forward.

The administrator saw her chance.

"Excellent! We have a new coach!"

To your astonishment, you saw that she was pointing directly at you. Parents, with relieved looks on their faces, turned to look at you. Some smirked. A few chuckled. All were joyful.

"Relax," one parent said. "The season doesn't start till next week."

"My kid's a shooter. You ought to see him shoot that ball. He's always been top scorer," another parent said as he gave you a good view of the bulldog tattooed on his bicep.

"My son plays small forward," another parent added, as if he bought his son the position from the National Basketball Association, which had granted the boy sole rights to play small forward on your team.

"I never knew you could coach, Dad," your son said as you walked to your car.

"Sure I can coach," you said. "How difficult can it be?" You hoped you at least *sounded* convincing.

Each winter, all across America, youth basketball leagues swing into action. Every year, thousands upon thousands of new coaches are tabbed to guide the players. The majority of those coaches have little or no experience coaching.

If you are one of those coaches, this book is for you. It is intended primarily for coaches of players from 6 to 12 years old, but it is applicable to coaches of older players as well. Use it as your rudder to guide you through your season. Use this book to

- Understand your role, and know what to expect, as a coach.
- Know the keys to being a good coach.
- Realize why kids play sports and consider how this should affect your approach to coaching.
- Bone up on the basic rules of basketball and learn how to impart those rules to your players.
- Provide for kids' safety and respond to emergency situations.

- Learn the general principles of teaching skills and tactics.
- Teach individual skills and team tactics.
- Coach effectively during games.
- Make the sport experience a meaningful and enjoyable one for the kids.
- Communicate effectively with parents, league administrators, referees, and players.
- Form positive alliances with parents, involving them in various ways.
- Plan for your season and your practices.
- Discover the keys to conducting productive practices.
- Celebrate victories and learn from defeats.
- Keep it all in perspective.

This guide presents the foundational concepts that effective coaches follow, and it shows you, step-by-step, how to incorporate those concepts, plan your season, and conduct your practices. It provides many forms you will need, including sample and blank season and practice plans, a sample letter to parents, an injury report and emergency information card, and a season evaluation form. It has games and drills you can use to teach your players the skills and tactics they need to know. It details how to execute the fundamental skills and tactics, so you will know what to teach—and it lays out *how* to teach. It is also replete with practical tips that will help your season be a success.

How This Book Is Organized

This book is organized in two parts. Part I covers coaching basics, and provides guidance in a number of areas, include your basic approach to coaching, communication keys, safety principles, and practice planning. Part II delves into the specifics of the skills and tactics your players will need to learn, ending with an entire chapter devoted to games and drills you can use to teach those skills and tactics.

Following Part II are six appendixes that you should find useful. This material includes a sample letter to parents, a medical emergency form, an injury report, blank season and practice plans you can use for your own planning, and a season evaluation form you can use at the end of your season.

Special Elements

Throughout the book you will find the following special elements:

caution

Cautions give you a loud "Heads up!" regarding issues or situations you want to avoid. These point out pitfalls, potential safety hazards, and any other items that could pose trouble to you or your team.

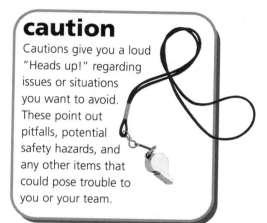

note

This is a note element. Notes give you relevant information that doesn't necessarily fit in the text flow.

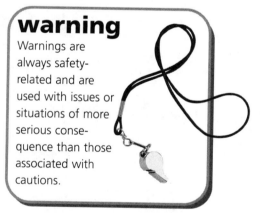

tip

Tips are given to help you do something more efficiently or to give you the "inside" view on how to accomplish something related to coaching basketball.

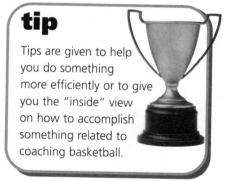

warning

Warnings are always safety-related and are used with issues or situations of more serious consequence than those associated with cautions.

PART 1

COACHING BASICS

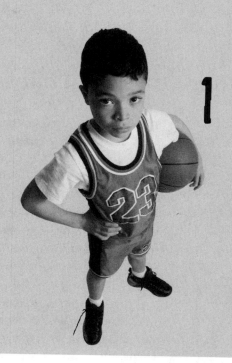

1

YOUR COACHING APPROACH

So you're a coach! Excellent. Most likely, you have a week or so to prepare for your first practice. But it's not time to jump into practice planning yet. Just as you will want your players to develop their fundamental skills first, you need to develop your basic coaching approach. Consider this chapter as your own personal coaching preparation. It provides the foundation for you to build upon.

Your Coaching Philosophy

Competition can bring out the best in us, and it can bring out the worst in us. You've read the stories of basketball brawls (generally at older levels of play, but youth levels are not immune to problems). You've probably witnessed parents in the stands screaming at the officials, at opposing players, or at their own kids. It doesn't happen all the time, but it happens often enough, even at the earliest levels of competition.

And it happens because of an overemphasis on winning. Our society places a premium on winning, and generally on winning at all costs. "Just win, baby," was the motto coined by Oakland Raiders owner Al Davis. This motto is fine at the professional level. It is *not* fine at the youth level. Why? Because when your focus is solely on winning, it comes at the expense of the kids you coach.

When your primary goal is to have an undefeated season or to win your league title, what happens? Every decision you make is based on whether it will help you win. So you play Colin, Seth, and Max, your least-skilled players, as little as your league rules allow. You try never to play them when the outcome is on the line. When they're in, you tell your team to "get the ball into the hands of the shooters," which translates into the lesser-skilled kids rarely touching the ball.

At the professional, collegiate, high school, and even upper youth levels, there's nothing wrong with this. At the lower youth levels, certainly at ages 6–12, plenty is wrong with it.

That overemphasis on winning comes at the cost of the kids' development, and of their love for the game. It results in low morale when players don't win enough games to meet your, or their parents', expectations. It certainly discourages the lesser-skilled players, who thought they were going to play a game but find that their main duty is to warm the bench and cheer on their teammates. It sends the message to kids that if they don't win, they have failed in their mission.

But their mission when they are 6–12 years old is to learn the game, to acquire and improve their skills, and to increase their understanding of the rules and tactics. It is not to pummel the opponent, to make a name for themselves in the local media, or to win every title in sight.

Your approach, then, should be to develop the whole player in these ways: physically, mentally, emotionally, and socially.

caution

Remember, the only way kids are going to improve their skills is by receiving good instruction and playing the game. At this level, that's your mission: to give everyone solid instruction, plenty of playing experience, and motivation to practice—not just with the team, but on their own as well.

Physical Development

It's your task as a coach to help your players acquire and develop the physical skills they need to perform. You need to teach them the basics: dribbling, passing, shooting, rebounding, playing defense, and so on.

In Chapter 6, "Player Development," you'll learn how to teach skills and tactics, and Chapters 9, "Offensive Skills and Tactics," and Chapter 10, "Defensive Skills and Tactics," are devoted to the correct execution of the skills and tactics you will be teaching, so you'll know step-by-step how to demonstrate proper execution.

Players' physical development is one of the obvious duties of a coach, and one that takes preeminence in practice. But practices and games can be used to develop players in other ways as well, including their mental development.

Mental Development

On defense, Jake loses his player, who cuts to the middle, comes off a screen to receive a pass, and makes an easy layup. On the way back down the court, you call out, "Watch the picks, you guys! Call out those screens!"

Basketball is fast-paced and ever-flowing. There are numerous players who are physically skilled—graceful, quick, strong, agile, coordinated—and they can perform the fundamental techniques just fine. But many of these players flounder on the court because they don't quite get what they're supposed to be doing at any one time, or they don't see a play developing or an opportunity opening up, or they don't understand the game's rules or the strategies involved.

Especially at the youth level, kids won't know all the rules and strategies of the game. If you teach skills in the context of how your players will use them in a game and tell them why they need to know how to perform the skill, chances are they will retain the *why* part. Also be aware that they might not understand these items the first few times you tell them, but as you continue to teach and remind them, it should sink in.

One of the greatest joys of coaching is seeing that your players know what to do in game situations. For example, they understand when to push the ball up the court on a fast break, when to double-team a player to force a turnover, and how to block out when the shot goes up.

This won't happen all at once, and much of it might not happen at all at the youngest levels. But if you clearly and simply explain the basic tactics and help your players understand the game and how to respond to various situations, they'll begin to get it. And their mental development is fun to watch. The mark of a good team, especially at the youth level, is not that they execute perfectly, but that they know what they should be trying to do in each situation.

Emotional Development

Each player is a unique person. Some players are outgoing; some are reserved. Some are excitable, and some laid-back. Some are jokers; some are serious. Some have the attention span of a gnat; others soak in most of what you say.

As a coach it is crucial that you understand that any one approach won't work the same with each child. Ben might be fine with some gentle kidding, whereas Alex might be bothered by the same kidding. Get to know your players as best you can in the first few weeks, and instruct and encourage them in the ways that will help them be ready and eager to learn and to play.

Remember that games produce situations that can become quite emotional for players (not to mention coaches!). Some players will be disconsolate after a loss; others won't be bothered at all. Help keep your players on an even keel. We talk more about how to do so in Chapter 7, "Game Time!"

Social Development

Basketball is great for social development. It takes a team effort to win. Players must rely on each other, pull for each other, and learn how to play with each other as they strive to win.

Use teachable moments to emphasize the team aspect of basketball. Such moments include the use of screens, a pick-and-roll, a give-and-go, double-teaming the player with the ball, or converting on a fast break. All involve teammates and all are executed for the good of the team.

Reinforce team unity in practices and at games. Don't treat "star" players differently. Look to enfold fringe players, those who are quiet or lesser-skilled and who might otherwise go unnoticed, in all team aspects. Also, be sure to emphasize the importance of everyone's contributions and point out those contributions when they happen.

Some Final Thoughts on Your Coaching Philosophy

Winning is a worthy goal, and one you should pursue as a team. However, as a youth basketball coach, winning cannot be the ultimate goal because the physical, mental, emotional, and social development of each player should be your ultimate goal.

When you develop your players' physical talents and mental abilities, you are putting

tip

Want to advise a player who has just made a mistake on the court? Then take him out—*after* he does something positive. Don't take a player out for making a mistake. Tell him how to correct his mistake, yes, but in an unobtrusive way, and include positive reinforcement as well.

them in a position to win. Teach them the game and its rules and tactics so they will be prepared to perform to the best of their abilities and knowledge. Encourage your players; let them know it's all right to make mistakes, and to learn from those mistakes.

When you focus on developing the whole player, that doesn't mean you're necessarily going to win your league or have a high winning percentage. It means you keep winning in its proper place—as a byproduct of sound player development, keeping each child's best interests at heart.

Sound difficult? It's not, if you develop the attributes of a good coach.

10 Attributes of a Good Coach

Just as your players are unique individuals, so are coaches. Maybe you're an extrovert; maybe you're an introvert. Maybe you're in a leadership position at work and are used to supervising people; maybe you have no supervisory experience at all. Regardless of your background, you can be an excellent youth basketball coach if you develop the following 10 attributes:

- Take your role seriously—but not *too* seriously.
- Be comfortable with being in charge.
- Be dependable and stable.
- Be patient.
- Be flexible.
- Enjoy getting to know your players.
- Desire to help kids learn and grow.
- Be an encourager.
- Be willing to learn.
- Have a sense of humor.

Let's take a brief look at each attribute.

Take Your Role Seriously

Now that you have volunteered to coach, commit yourself to the time and energy it will take to coach. Showing up on time at the practice court or for the game is not enough. Show up prepared to conduct the practice, prepared to coach your players during the game, and ready to instruct and supervise your players. Your role is to teach your players how to play basketball. They're looking to learn from you.

On the other hand, keep things in their proper perspective. These are games, learning experiences—hopefully *fun* experiences—for kids who are 6–12 years old. Their basketball experiences generally *are* fun, win or lose, unless they are tarnished by overzealous coaches or parents who place such great emphasis on winning that all the fun drains out of the game.

Keep the fun in the game. Keep the kids' best interests at heart. Relax, take a deep breath, enjoy the moment, and focus on the task at hand, such as how to make a good bounce pass, how to block out, or how to play good team defense.

Use your players as a guide. If they look tense, are unusually quiet at practice, or they're avoiding your look, they're probably taking their cues from you, and you had better ease up. On the other hand, if they're cracking jokes and goofing off and aren't focusing on the task at hand, you need to gain control. You'll learn some tips on how to do so in Chapter 5, "Practice Plans."

Ultimately, what you're after is a steady pace at practice where learning and fun are synonymous and ongoing.

Be Comfortable with Being in Charge

Every child will be looking to you for instruction. You have to be comfortable with being the leader, the teacher, and the resident expert who knows how to instruct and conduct effective practices. You need to know what your goal is in each practice, and you need to steer your kids in that direction while maintaining an open and friendly atmosphere within that context.

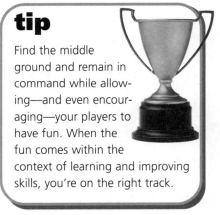

tip

Find the middle ground and remain in command while allowing—and even encouraging—your players to have fun. When the fun comes within the context of learning and improving skills, you're on the right track.

If you're not comfortable being in charge and are unable to set the proper tone for practice, one of two things happens: either the practice crumbles into chaos and nothing is learned as kids misbehave and don't pay attention, or you overreact to a little goofing off and rule with severe authority.

Be Dependable and Stable

Be on time at every practice and game, and be there ready to execute your plan. If you can't make a game or practice, alert your assistant coach or a parent who is willing and able to take over.

The kids are counting on you. When they know they can rely on you to be there and be ready, that lets them focus on learning, practicing, and performing. When the kids know you respond evenly and fairly in all situations, they feel free to practice without worrying about how you might respond to a turnover or a missed shot. Coaches who are dependable and stable create a healthy learning environment for their players.

Be Patient

If you're a parent, you know the value of patience. It can be difficult enough raising a couple of young kids. When you have 10–12 youngsters at your charge, patience is at a premium.

They won't pay attention to your every word. They won't always understand your instruction on the first, or second or third, try. They will make the same types of mistakes over and over. They will ask you goofy questions and act, well, like the kids they are. They will, in short, try your patience. If you don't have a lot, here's your chance to develop this virtue.

Don't expect perfection, either in game-time performance or practice-time behavior. Let the kids know what you expect of them, in terms of their behavior and their listening to your directives. Also keep in mind what the goal is for the day, whether you're at a practice or a game, and steer the ship in that direction. When you guide your players with patient resolve, your practices will be more effective.

Don't mistake being patient with letting your players do whatever they want to do. Don't tolerate inappropriate words or actions. Step in and correct players in these situations. Just remember to be patient as they strive to learn how to shoot, pass, dribble, defend, and rebound.

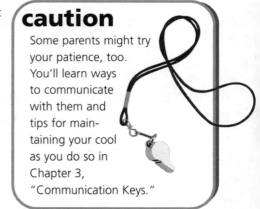

caution

Some parents might try your patience, too. You'll learn ways to communicate with them and tips for maintaining your cool as you do so in Chapter 3, "Communication Keys."

Be Flexible

Being flexible is another hallmark of a good coach. You might have worked out your season plan, in terms of what you want to teach and when you want to teach it, but you might have to adjust that schedule if the kids haven't picked up the requisite skills yet. For example, it's no use teaching your 10-year-olds how to execute a pick-and-roll if they are having trouble simply dribbling and passing.

You have to constantly assess how your players are doing, what they need to learn next, and what they have been able to master at least well enough to move on to something new. It's good to work out a season plan in advance; just be ready to adjust that plan along the way.

Enjoy Getting to Know Your Players

Hopefully you enjoy being around kids, or you wouldn't have volunteered to coach. The best coaches appreciate kids for who they are and want to help them develop their skills and learn a sport. These coaches understand that their players are full-fledged children, not miniature adults. And these coaches enjoy being around their players. They can see the game from their players' perspectives while maintaining their adult view and their authority as a coach. They appreciate each child for his own unique personality and skills.

With that in mind, realize that the approach that works with Justin, who is effusive and outgoing, might not work with Sam, who is quiet and reflective. Learn to communicate with players on an individual level. Pay attention to what each player responds best to, and develop a rapport with each child that will help him learn and grow best.

That doesn't mean you should change your personality to suit each player. It means you should be aware of each child's distinct personality and relate to him as an individual.

Getting to know your players on an individual level is one of the joys of coaching. By doing so, you can tune into their needs as players and more readily help them develop their skills.

Desire to Help Kids Learn and Grow

It's late in a tight ballgame, you're down by two points, and your point guard, Kevin, is dribbling near the top of the key. A teammate flashes open in the middle, and as Kevin is about to pass the ball, it is stolen by a defender who takes it the length of the court and scores. Now you're four points down with time dwindling. You call a timeout.

You have a couple of choices at this point:

- You could chew out Kevin in front of the other players for his boneheaded play, shouting that you've gone over and over how he has to protect the ball and be aware of what's going on, adding that if he had hit his teammate with a pass, you would be tied right now.

- You could tell Kevin to let it go, to not let it bother him, and to keep his head in the game. Remind him of the positive ways he has already contributed. Then you could tell your players what you want them to do in the waning moments. This might include giving the ball back to Kevin to penetrate, if he has the confidence to do so.

Hopefully, you would choose the latter. You're more likely to do so if your focus is on helping the players learn and grow. This is really what coaching is all about at the youth level. It's very satisfying to watch your players acquire new skills, learn the game's tactics, and be able to execute plays more consistently. These things happen when your central desire as a coach is to help them learn and grow.

Be an Encourager

Good instruction is the seed and encouragement is the water that helps the seed grow. Your players need your encouragement as they attempt to learn the physical and mental skills it takes to play basketball. You'll learn more about specific ways to encourage your players in Chapter 3.

Be Willing to Learn

Just as your players will be learning throughout the season how to play the game, you'll be learning how to coach. There are many ways you can learn:

note

One of the greatest things you can do as a coach is to motivate your players to practice on their own. Practice and game time is limited, but all kids need is a ball, a goal, and motivation to practice and improve on their own. It's often this solitary or informal practice time that contributes significantly to their development throughout the season.

- **Through this book**—Use this guide to shape your approach to coaching and to formulate your season and practice plans.

- **Through your own experience**—Know that you'll make some mistakes along the way. That's okay. Be willing to learn from your mistakes. You'll discover, through experience, what works for you and what doesn't. You might also find that what works well for you this year might not work as well next year with different players.

- **Through observing other coaches**—You can learn from both good and bad coaches. What sets good coaches apart from ones who aren't so good? How do they communicate with their players, and *what* do they communicate? How do they behave on the bench? How do they relate with officials, and what kind of coaching do they do during the game? How do their players conduct themselves during and after the game? You can learn a lot through observation. Put to use what works for you, and model yourself after competent and caring coaches.

- **Through coaching clinics**—If your league offers a coaching clinic, attend it. If not, keep your eye out for coaching clinics in your area. You can often pick up some pointers and make helpful contacts at these clinics.

Most importantly, be willing to learn to coach. Many former players rely solely on their playing experience to inform their coaching. With that same thinking, you might assume that because you've had experience sitting in a dentist's chair and having a tooth drilled, you are qualified to pick up a dentist's drill and go to work in someone's mouth.

Playing and coaching call on a different set of skills. Having playing experience can help you as a coach in many ways, but it doesn't take the place of knowing how to coach. This book will help you develop your coaching skills.

Have a Sense of Humor

Enjoy your time as a coach. Basketball is meant to be fun. Your intent as a coach shouldn't be to "entertain the troops," but there's nothing wrong with a little natural levity. It's okay to laugh and joke with your players; you can do this while still moving forward with your instruction.

Just make sure your humor doesn't come at the expense of someone else—even an opponent. Don't make fun of someone's mistake, but do enjoy lighthearted moments as they come up.

> **caution**
>
> Having fun and being friendly with the kids doesn't mean you should try to be buddies with them. They're not looking for a new friend; they're looking for a coach to help them learn the game.

Don't use humor when kids need instruction, but do use it to diffuse tension. For example, if Jimmy is about to go to the free throw line with your team down by three points late in the game, and he asks what he should do, don't say, "Make both free throws, and then steal the inbounds pass and score on that, too." Jimmy's not asking for a joke, but for a little help. He'd be better-served if you told him, "Just keep your focus. Get in your rhythm, relax, and shoot. You can do it."

10 Keys to Being a Good Coach

We've just gone over the attributes of a good coach. If you have those attributes, or can develop them, you're on your way to being a good coach. But some other key elements to coaching extend beyond these basic characteristics. When you exhibit the traits we talked about in the previous section and possess the 10 keys we present in this section, you'll excel.

What are the keys to good coaching? To be a good basketball coach, you must

- Know the basics of the sport.
- Plan for your season and practices.
- Conduct effective practices.
- Teach skills and tactics.
- Correct players in a way that helps them improve.
- Teach and model good sporting behavior.
- Provide for safety.
- Communicate effectively with players, parents, officials, and league administrators.

- Coach effectively during games.
- Know what constitutes success in youth basketball.

Let's look at each of these keys in a little more depth.

Know the Basics of the Sport

You can't teach what you don't know. You need to be prepared to teach your players the basic rules, the skills, and the tactics of basketball. Especially at the younger ages, this information is quite basic, but that doesn't mean you automatically know all you need to know.

The next chapter covers the basic rules and Chapters 9 and 10 cover the skills and tactics you need to know and teach. Be sure you know the rules, skills, and tactics before your season begins.

Plan for Your Season and Practices

You can know all you need to know about the rules, skills, and tactics, but if you don't have a game plan for when and how to teach them, you—and, more importantly, your players—will be in trouble.

Planning doesn't mean thinking about a drill you might run that day as you drive to practice. It means considering the big picture for the entire season and breaking that picture down into individual practice plans so you're prepared for every practice. You'll learn how to create season and practice plans in Chapter 5.

Conduct Effective Practices

When you have a practice plan in hand, you are on your way to conducting an effective practice. But there's a big difference between having a plan and being able to execute it. Two coaches could have the exact same practice plan, and the experiences could be vastly different for their players, depending on how the coaches execute that plan. In Chapter 5, you'll learn the keys to conducting effective practices.

Teach Skills and Tactics

This, of course, is one of your primary duties. Your ability to teach skills and tactics will significantly impact your players' development. Remember, the abilities to *perform* and to *teach* are different abilities. So, if you've played before, don't assume your playing experience will make you a great teacher. Rather, learn how to be an effective teacher. In Chapter 6, you'll learn the keys to teaching skills and tactics.

Correct Players in a Way That Helps Them Improve

If one of your players makes the same mistake repeatedly, it might be he's simply unable to perform the skill yet—or it might be you haven't helped him understand *how* to correct his faulty technique. Part of being an effective teacher is being able to observe your players' performances, detect mechanical and tactical errors, and help them correct those errors. In Chapter 6, you'll learn how to detect and correct flaws and help your players improve their skills.

Teach and Model Good Sporting Behavior

Your players will take their cues from you, not only on how to play the game, but also in how to behave at games. Behave responsibly and treat all involved with respect. Leave the arguing and gamesmanship for NBA and college coaches. You'll learn more on modeling good behavior in Chapter 7.

Provide for Players' Safety

This is one of your most important duties. You'll need to know how to conduct safe practices and how to respond to injuries when they occur. Chapter 4, "Safety Principles," is devoted to this topic.

Communicate Effectively

You'll do a lot of communicating as a coach, primarily with your players, but also with their parents, officials, other coaches, and league administrators. You might know exactly how to block out to rebound, but if you don't know how to communicate how to do so, your players probably won't understand the mechanics involved. Chapter 3 explains how to communicate effectively, and what needs to be communicated and to whom, in a variety of situations.

Coach Effectively During Games

There's a difference between coaching at practice and coaching during games. The goals are different, and what you communicate is different. You'll learn about those differences, and the keys to coaching effectively during games, in Chapter 7.

Know What Success Is

By now you should have the idea that success at the youth level isn't based on your winning percentage. Rather, it's based on your ability to develop your players' skills and help them maintain their enthusiasm for the game, and on many other factors. Winning is an important and worthy goal, but you can have a successful season no matter what your record is. In Chapter 8, "Ingredients of a Successful

Season," you'll learn what makes a season *truly* successful, and you'll also learn how to gauge your success.

Final Thoughts on the Keys to Being a Good Coach

When you use these 10 keys as the foundation of your coaching, you'll be successful. In fact, learning how to use these keys is what the rest of Part I, "Coaching Basics," is all about.

What to Expect As a Coach

The dream of youth league coaches goes something like this:

- All their players show up on time for every practice.
- The players pay attention every minute.
- The players soak in the instruction and acquire the physical skills and tactical knowledge with ease.
- The players perform like seasoned veterans from game one.
- The parents are enthusiastic, supportive, and appreciative of the coach's efforts and ability to bring the team together.
- After winning the league championship, the players are somehow able to hoist the coach up on their scrawny shoulders and the parents roar their approval.
- To cap everything off, one rich parent throws a victory party at an expensive steak house, and during the party the teary-eyed parents come by, one by one, to thank the coach for making such a difference in their son's or daughter's life.

Conversely, the nightmare of youth league coaches goes something like this:

- You have to call all your players the night before the first practice because the league switched your practice court at the last moment.
- Not all the players assigned to your team show up for the first practice.
- The time you meant to take to plan for the season and the first practice evaporated, and you feel rushed and unprepared.
- About half the kids on your team have never played basketball before.
- A couple of kids are uncooperative.
- Another kid sprains his ankle in the first practice.
- At the first game, you have your playing rotation figured out, but three players don't show up, so you have to rearrange everything at the last moment.
- You find that two fathers are more than willing to shout helpful coaching tips to you, while a mother in the stands critiques the official all game long.

- After the game, a couple of parents complain about where you played their kids, or how much playing time they received.
- Your calls to the league administrator are never returned.

Hopefully that nightmare won't be your reality. But the point is this: Be prepared for anything. Know that mundane, tedious, and sometimes bothersome things will infiltrate your season.

Expect to be tested, in some ways by your players, in others by their parents. Expect the officiating to be less than perfect. Expect your players to make mistakes, and expect some of them to be upset by those mistakes. Expect some parents to be very supportive, others to be seemingly nonexistent, and a few to present challenging situations. Expect the unexpected, and know that not all things will go according to your plan.

Keep your focus on what's best for the kids, and base all your decisions on that. That's why it's so important to develop the attributes of a good coach. When you are patient, flexible, dependable, and comfortable with being in charge, you can handle any situation that comes your way.

What Is Expected of *You* As a Coach

What is expected of you is summed up in the keys to good coaching:

- You are expected to know the basics of basketball, its rules, its strategies, and the skills involved.
- You are expected to be prepared to coach—to plan for the season and for practices—so that there is a logical cohesiveness to your instruction, a purpose for each practice, and a sense of moving forward throughout the season, with the players always learning and always improving.
- You are expected to be able to teach the skills and tactics of basketball, explain when and how the skill or tactic is used, and demonstrate how to execute it. (If you are unable to adequately demonstrate it, you can use an assistant coach or a volunteer parent to do so.)
- You are expected to observe your players as they practice the skills and tactics to detect what they are doing incorrectly and to help them make corrections.
- You are expected to model good sporting behavior; communicate appropriately with players, parents, officials, and the opposition; and show respect for all involved.
- You are expected to teach your players how to win with class without rubbing it in or taunting their opponents, and how to lose with dignity, learning from the loss and making neither a win nor a loss bigger than it is.

- You are expected to conduct practices as safely as possible, providing direct supervision at all times, conducting drills and games that are safe, warning players about inherent dangers, and instituting team rules that promote safety.

- You are expected to know how to coach during games, doing what's appropriate and best for your players' development and conducting yourself appropriately.

- Finally, you are expected to keep in mind what constitutes success in youth basketball. You are striving to win your games, of course, but far greater than that, you are giving your players opportunities to develop their skills, to have fun, to compete, to play together as a team, and to get the most of their abilities. They are there to grow, learn, and develop, and that development is your main task.

Now, not all parents or players will have these expectations. Some will be focused only on winning and become frustrated if your coaching decisions don't reflect the same outlook. In Chapter 3, you'll learn when and how to communicate with players and parents who have these expectations.

It's important that you keep these expectations in mind throughout the season. They will act as your rudder, guiding you through any choppy waters you might experience.

Equipment and Insurance

Check with your league regarding equipment they issue each team and insurance they might carry. In many cases, the league provides balls and pinneys for each team, and it's your responsibility to keep and maintain the equipment and return it at season's end. In addition, if you want to keep statistics, you should have a scorebook for your games.

In some cases, insurance is provided through a coaching certification program or a league; in other cases, it's not provided. Some leagues carry insurance policies that cover all teams and participants involved, including coaches and officials. If insurance is an important issue for you, talk to your league administrator about it.

Last, But Not Least: Why Kids Play Basketball

Kids play basketball for a lot of reasons. Many have grand dreams of being the next LeBron James or Kevin Garnett or Allen Iverson. Some play for negative reasons, such as their parents pushing them into it. Their father might be trying to relive his faded dreams of stardom. Or they might have chosen basketball over a less desirable activity, such as taking tuba lessons.

But the overwhelming majority play for positive reasons. Those reasons are

- They want to have fun.
- They want to hang out with their friends.
- They want to develop their abilities.
- They like the excitement of sports.
- They want to be part of a winning effort.

That order is not random; it reflects the most common responses kids give when they are asked for the main reasons they play basketball.

Notice that *fun* is at the top of the list, and *winning* is at the bottom. Winning is important to them, but not nearly as important as it is to have fun and be with their friends.

What does this mean for you? It means you should focus on fun and development throughout the season and you should strive to win, but not at the expense of fun and development. It's that simple. And you'll be amazed at how well your players perform when they're having fun and developing their skills.

THE ABSOLUTE MINIMUM

This chapter introduced you to the basic concepts of coaching basketball. You learned about your coaching approach, the attributes of a good coach, the keys to being a good coach, what you should expect as a coach, what is expected of you as a coach, and why kids play basketball. Keep these points in mind:

- Base your coaching approach on the players' fun and development. Always keep their overall development in mind.
- Keep the attributes of a good coach front and center. When you approach your coaching with these traits in mind, you are bound to be successful.
- Plan your practices. Learn how to teach skills and tactics and how to correct mistakes.
- Expect the unexpected, and be guided by your coaching approach in all situations.
- Live up to your own expectations, based on the keys to good coaching.
- Understand that kids play basketball to have fun, to be with their friends, and to develop their skills.

Coaching with these things in mind will help you plan and implement a fun and constructive basketball season that produces enjoyment and plenty of learning!

2

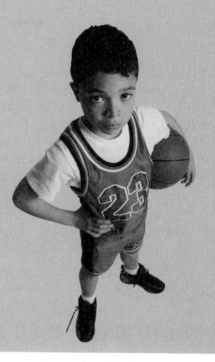

RULES OF THE GAME

Basketball has some basic rules that even the most casual fan knows:

- A field goal is worth two points (and, in some cases, three).
- A free throw is worth one point.
- You can't plow over your opponent.
- If the ball goes out of bounds, it goes to the team that didn't touch it last.
- You can't run with the ball; you have to dribble it, pass it, or shoot it.

There are a host of rules your players need to be aware of, and as their coach, it's your duty to teach them those rules. What's blocking, and what's charging? What's a backcourt violation? What does it mean to "double dribble?" What is traveling, and when is a player called for it? What does the bonus situation refer to, and when does it occur?

In addition to the basic rules, you have to know the modified rules of your league and relay those modifications to your players. Many rules are modified to make the game more appropriate for younger players. For example, youth leagues lower the basket so kids can practice good shooting form and have a better chance of making shots. The size of the court is diminished, the length of the game is shorter, the ball size is smaller, and the free throw distance is shorter for youth league play. Check with your league administrator to learn which modified rules your league has in place.

Although your primary duty is to teach your players the skills they need to perform well, they need to understand the context within which they'll perform those skills, and the rules provide part of that context.

In this chapter you'll learn about the basic rules so you can prepare your players to know what is allowed on offense and on defense.

Basic Youth Basketball Rules

The following is meant to be a primer for the basics, not the final word on every rule in complete detail. The rules in this section are divided into five categories:

- Court, equipment, and time
- Players
- Scoring
- Fouls
- Violations

Court, Equipment, and Time

As mentioned, the court dimensions are smaller for youth leagues. The court is divided into two halves. When the offense is on their side of the court (the side on which they shoot), that's called the *frontcourt;* the opposite end is called the *backcourt.* (Note that similar terminology is also used to refer to players. Frontcourt players are the bigger players—the center and typically the two forwards. Backcourt players refer to the two guards.) See Figure 2.1 for court markings and terminology. As we go through the chapter, you'll learn about certain rules that pertain to particular portions of the court.

The basket is mounted on a backboard and is generally seven, eight, or nine feet high for youth play, depending on the age. The ball used in league play is typically made of leather and is smaller than regulation size (a size five or six ball instead of the regulation size seven). The league chooses the ball size. It's a good idea to have your players practice with the league-size ball, both at practice and at home, so they get the feel for the size of ball they will be handling during games.

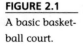

FIGURE 2.1

A basic basketball court.

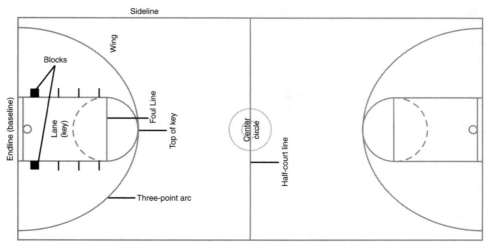

League game length varies, depending on the age and on the particular rules for that league. Some leagues run a *continuous clock* (meaning the clock does not stop when the ball goes out of bounds or for any other action that normally would stop the clock). Others run a continuous clock but allow teams to take a certain number of timeouts per half, during which the clock stops. Other leagues might run a *regulation clock*, albeit shorter, meaning the clock stops when the ball goes out of bounds, when a player is fouled, when a violation is committed, and so on.

Youth league games generally run from 24 to 32 minutes, played in either quarters or halves.

Players

Five players for each team are on the court at one time. The position terminology varies a bit. Often, but not always, a team has one center or post player, two forwards, and two guards. A common way to refer to the players is by position:

- #1—Point guard
- #2—Shooting guard
- #3—Small forward
- #4—Power forward
- #5—Post player or center

The *center* generally is your tallest or biggest player and plays down low near the basket to take advantage of her height. The center is also called the *post* because that describes the area she's often in. The post positions are along the foul line, leading from the free throw line to the basket. It's called *high post* if she's out near the free throw line, and *low post* if she's down in the blocks near the basket (see Figure 2.2). Much of the center's action is within 10 feet of the basket.

FIGURE 2.2

Low post and
high post
positions.

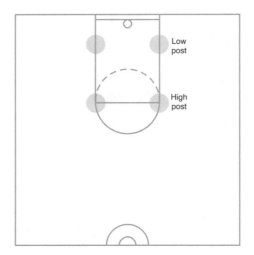

Forwards are generally taller than guards but shorter than the center. Forwards typi-cally cover more ground than the center; they roam down low, run the baseline, and move out to the wing position (refer to Figure 2.1). Most of their action is within 10 to 15 feet of the basket.

Forwards often are better outside shooters than the center, and perhaps a little quicker or more agile. They need to be able to cut, move, feint, get open, and block out for rebounds. Some kids enjoy mixing it up under the boards, going for rebounds, while others shy away from it. You want your forwards to be hungry for the ball, to enjoy going after it aggressively while being under control.

Guards are typically the smallest players on the court. They often are the quickest players as well, and benefit from good ball-handling skills because they usually bring the ball up the court and run the offense. They often shoot from far-ther out, and thus need to refine their outside shots. Perhaps even more importantly, they need to have good "court sense," seeing plays unfold and knowing how to move the ball so their team gets a good scoring opportunity.

note

Many teams today use a *motion offense* in which all five players handle the ball, post up, shoot from outside, and penetrate. They play on the perimeter and con-tinually move, using post, for-ward, and guard skills. A motion offense might be a good one for you to consider for your team, if your players can handle the ball well.

Often a team has a *point guard* and a *shooting guard*. The point guard brings the ball up the court and does much of the initial ball handling; this guard is your best ball-handler and passer. The shooting guard often plays in the wing area and is one of your best shooters on the team.

Scoring

Some youth leagues play with a three-point rule, in which baskets made beyond the three-point line (refer to Figure 2.1) are worth three points. When this rule is not in effect, baskets made beyond the three-point arc count for two points. All baskets made inside the three-point arc count for two points.

If the three-point rule is in effect, no part of the shooter's feet can be touching the court on or inside the three-point line before the shooter releases the shot (for a basket to count as a three-pointer). After the shot is released, a made basket counts as three points even if the player's feet land inside the three-point arc, so long as they were behind the line when the shot went up.

A team is awarded one point for every made free throw. At lower levels, some leagues don't shoot free throws, even if fouls occur on shots. Instead, they award the ball out of bounds to the team that was fouled.

Fouls

A *personal foul* occurs when a player makes illegal contact with an opponent. This illegal contact can happen in a variety of ways, for example

- *Blocking* occurs when a defender illegally impedes an offensive player's progress. If a defender's feet are not set and contact is made, blocking will be called.

- Charging is a *player control foul* (the player in control of the ball committed the foul). A *charge* is illegal contact by the ball handler, who charges into a defensive player, usually during a drive to the basket. If a defender's feet are set and he is stationary before contact is made, charging will be called. Charging can also be called if the defender's feet are not set but the dribbler drives into the defender's torso.

- A *flagrant foul* is a violent and intentional foul; for example, kneeing, kicking, or punching.

- *Hand-checking* is illegal use of a defender's hands on the offensive player, to impede the player's progress. This occurs when the offensive player is in front of the defender.

- *Holding* is called when a player holds on to and restricts an opponent's movement.

- An *illegal screen* occurs when the player setting the screen is moving when she contacts an opposing player.

- An *intentional foul* happens when a player intentionally fouls another player. An example is when a defender doesn't go for the ball, but intentionally commits a foul to ensure that a basket is not scored.

- An *offensive foul* is one committed by any offensive player, either with or without the ball. When it's committed by the player with the ball, it's called charging. When the foul is committed by the player with the ball, no foul shots are awarded. When committed by a player away from the ball, foul shots are awarded if the number of team fouls is over the limit.

- *Over the back* is called when a player makes contact from behind with an opponent who is going for a rebound.

- *Pushing* is illegally using the hands or body to impede the progress of an opponent.

- *Reaching in* is a foul committed by a defender trying to steal the ball or knock it away from the ball handler. When defenders reach for the ball, they can't make contact with the ball handler's body.

- *Tripping* is called when a player uses a leg or foot to cause an opponent to stumble or fall. Tripping doesn't have to be intentional to be called.

In addition, a referee can call a *technical foul* on any player, coach, or team personnel. This foul does not involve contact while the ball is live. Examples of when technical fouls would be called are when a player uses foul language, unsporting conduct, obscene gestures, or throws the ball in anger.

What happens after a foul depends on the type of foul and the situation. See the sidebar "Consequences of Fouls."

CONSEQUENCES OF FOULS

There are three categories of fouls to consider: shooting fouls; personal fouls; and technical, intentional, or flagrant fouls.

- **Shooting fouls**—If a player is fouled in the act of shooting and the ball goes in, the basket counts and the player gets one free throw. If a player is fouled in the act of shooting and the ball does not go in, the player is awarded two free throws. If the three-point rule is in effect and the shooter is fouled behind the three-point arc, he gets three free throws.

- **Personal fouls**—If a player is fouled while not in the act of shooting and his team is not in the bonus situation, the team that was fouled gets the ball out of bounds. If the team is in the bonus, the player who was fouled gets a one-and-one free throw opportunity. If he makes the first free throw, he is awarded a second free throw. If he misses the first free throw, the ball is live and no additional free throw is given.

  The *bonus situation* simply means that a team has committed a certain number of fouls in a half (this number is determined by the league). After that number has been committed, the opponent is in the bonus, and any nonshooting foul through the rest of that half will send the opponent to the line for a one-and-one opportunity. In many youth leagues, after a few more fouls are committed after the bonus has been reached, two free throws are awarded for any foul thereafter.

■ **Technical, intentional, or flagrant fouls**—Two free throws are awarded to the opponent, and the player who was fouled shoots the free throws (except in the case of a technical foul; any of the five players on the court can shoot the free throws). The team that shot the free throws then gets the ball out of bounds to resume play.

Violations

A *violation* happens when a player or a team violates a rule, resulting in the ball being turned over to the opponent. Here are brief explanations of common violations:

■ A *backcourt violation* occurs when the team with the ball is unable to get the ball into its frontcourt within 10 seconds after passing the ball inbounds.

■ *Carrying* or *palming* the ball is called when the dribbler carries the ball at the top of her dribble—that is, the ball rests briefly on her hand before she turns her hand over again and dribbles.

■ A *closely-guarded violation* occurs if the player with the ball holds the ball, dribbles while remaining stationary, or dribbles horizontally for more than five seconds while being closely guarded.

■ *Double dribble* can happen in two ways. The dribbler uses both hands on the ball at the same time to dribble, or the player dribbles, stops dribbling, and then dribbles again.

■ A *lane violation* occurs when an offensive player, either with or without the ball, is in the free throw lane for three consecutive seconds.

■ *Over and back* is called when the team with the ball in its frontcourt has the ball go into the backcourt, and the last player to touch the ball in the frontcourt was an offensive player. (It's not over and back if a defender knocks the ball into the backcourt; in that case, the ball is live and either team can recover it.)

■ A *shot clock violation* happens if the team with the ball does not get off a shot that hits the rim before the shot-clock buzzer goes off. The ball must leave the shooter's hand before the buzzer goes off, and it must subsequently hit the rim.

■ *Throw-in violations* occur in two situations: The player passing the ball inbounds takes more than five seconds to release the ball after the referee has started his count, or the player passing the ball inbounds does not keep a pivot foot on the floor until she releases the ball. Players must maintain a pivot foot in all inbounds situations except for those occurring after made field goals or free throws.

■ *Traveling* is called when the ball handler moves both feet without dribbling.

How the Game Is Played

You've been introduced to the basics of the game, in terms of rules involving players, scoring, fouls, and violations. Here you learn the rudiments of how the game is played—that is, the general parameters that guide it from beginning to end.

A center jump begins play, with the referee tossing the ball up in the center circle between two players, one from each team. Each player tries to tip the ball to one of her teammates.

The team in possession moves the ball legally into its frontcourt, by either dribbling or passing, and maneuvers for a good shot. The consequences of various fouls were covered earlier in this chapter; if a team commits a violation, the ball is turned over to the opponent.

> **note**
>
> Realize that many violations are either not called or are modified to be appropriate for the age and skill levels of the players. For example, an extra step might be allowed before traveling is called, or one double dribble per possession might be allowed before calling a violation. Check with your league on violation modifications.

If a player makes a field goal, the offense is awarded two points (or three points, if the field goal was a valid three-point attempt and a three-point rule is in place). A team scores one point for each free throw its players make.

After a made basket, the player passing the ball inbounds can run the baseline, staying behind the baseline and out of bounds, and must release the ball within five seconds. The offense then has 10 seconds to get the ball into its frontcourt. From there, the offense sets up to get a good shot. Any missed shot can be rebounded by either team.

Coaches can substitute players according to their league rules. Sometimes substitutes can enter only when the ball is dead and they are beckoned on by the referee. Some leagues allow substitutions "on the fly," with a substitute entering the game when the ball is live and the player being subbed for exiting immediately. Check with your league on this and all modifications.

The team that scores the most points wins. If the game is tied at the end of regulation, generally an overtime period is played to determine the winner.

Terms

The following terms should help you become familiar with the language, rules, and situations you will encounter as you coach your team. I won't repeat definitions that have been given earlier in this chapter.

- **Alternating possession**—Rather than use a jump ball to start the second half or to resume play after a *held ball* (see below), teams alternate possessions in these instances. So, if Team A wins the jump ball to begin the game,

Team B gets the next alternating possession, whether that's through a held ball or to begin the second half.

- **Backcourt**—The half of the court that includes the defensive team's basket. (Backcourt players refer to guards or perimeter players.)
- **Dribble**—To bounce the ball on the floor.
- **Free throw**—A shot taken from behind the free throw line as the result of a foul.
- **Frontcourt**—The half of the court that includes the offensive team's basket. (Frontcourt players refer to big players underneath the basket.)
- **Held ball**—A ball that is jointly held by a player from each team.
- **Incidental contact**—This is contact between two opponents in which neither player is restricted in movement or when they are in equally favorable positions and they make contact, such as in going for a loose ball. No foul is called for incidental contact.
- **Jump ball**—A jump ball begins the game. From there on, held balls result in the ball being awarded based on the alternating possession rule.
- **Pass**—A pass is made by throwing the ball.
- **Pivot**—A pivot refers to one foot of the ball handler. At least one foot must remain in the same spot on the floor unless the ball handler is dribbling, passing, or shooting the ball. The player may turn on that pivot foot so long as the foot does not move from that spot.
- **Player-to-player defense**—This is a system of defense in which each player is assigned to guard one specific opponent, no matter where that opponent is on the court.
- **Rebound**—When a shot is missed, the player who gains possession of the ball does so by rebounding it.
- **Screen**—A screen, also called a *pick,* is set by a stationary player who stands in the way of a teammate's defender. The teammate brushes past the screener, and in doing so is able to break free from her defender.
- **Steal**—A steal happens when a defender legally gains possession of the ball from the player she is guarding.
- **Zone defense**—This is a system of defense in which each player is assigned a specific portion of the court. That player is responsible for whatever action happens in that portion of the court.

Signals

Signals are one way that referees communicate with coaches, players, other game officials, and fans. Following are common basketball signals you should become familiar with. Figure 2.3 has to do with clock situations, Figure 2.4 deals with scoring issues, and Figure 2.5 illustrates various fouls and violations.

note

Many volunteer referees aren't used to signaling and haven't been trained to use signals. If you're unclear of a call, find a reasonable way to ask the referee to clarify her call.

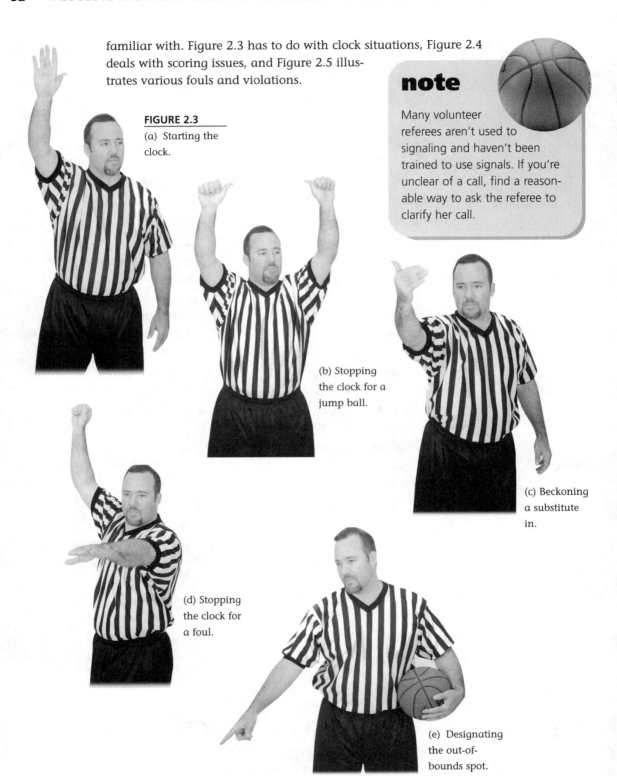

FIGURE 2.3

(a) Starting the clock.

(b) Stopping the clock for a jump ball.

(c) Beckoning a substitute in.

(d) Stopping the clock for a foul.

(e) Designating the out-of-bounds spot.

FIGURE 2.4

(a) Scoring one point.

(b) Scoring two points.

(c) Scoring three points.

(d) Three-point attempt.

(e) No score.

(f) Bonus situation.

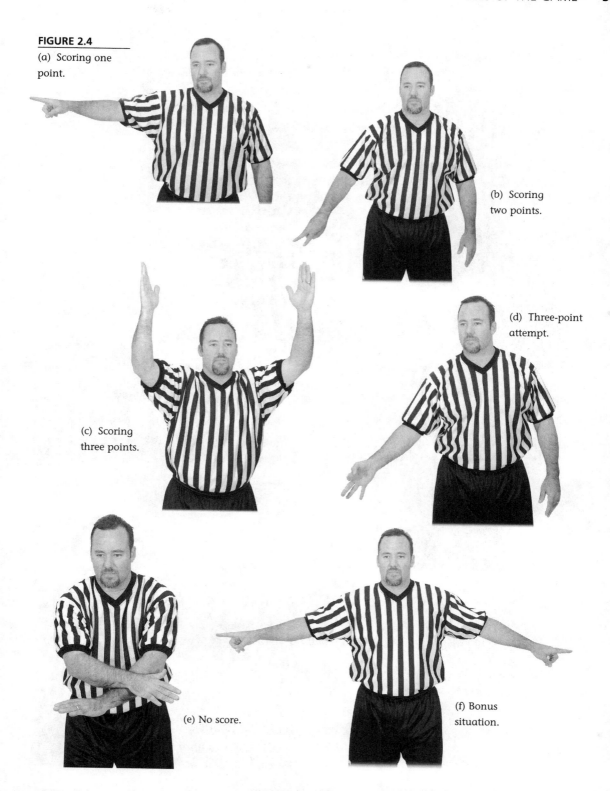

FIGURE 2.5

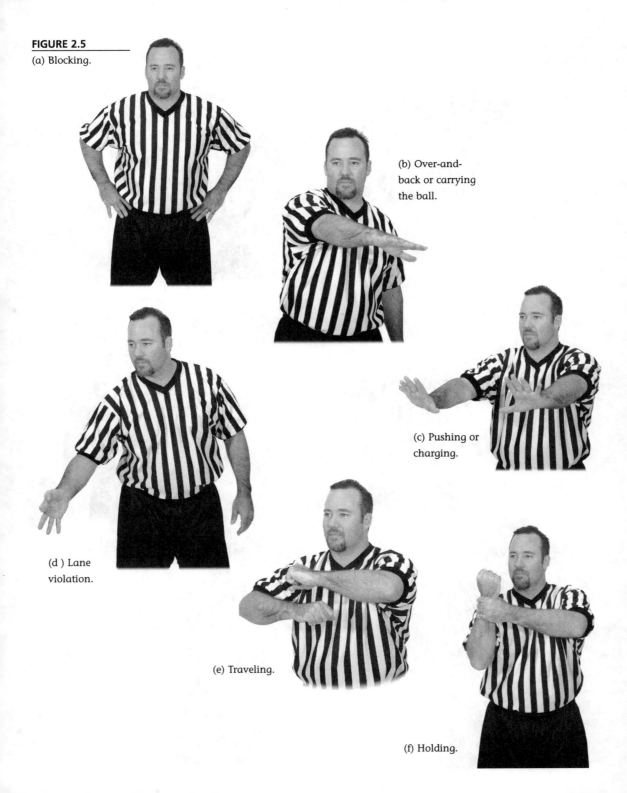

(a) Blocking.

(b) Over-and-back or carrying the ball.

(c) Pushing or charging.

(d) Lane violation.

(e) Traveling.

(f) Holding.

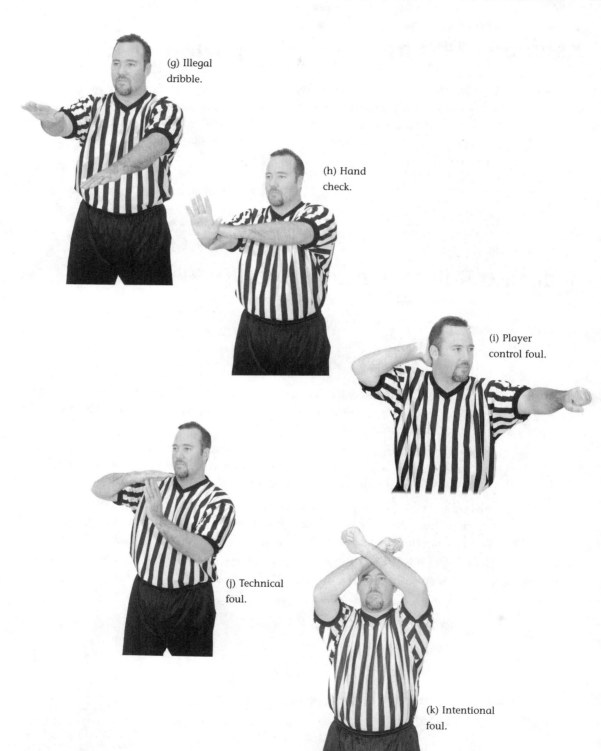

(g) Illegal dribble.

(h) Hand check.

(i) Player control foul.

(j) Technical foul.

(k) Intentional foul.

Keep on Learning

Knowing the rules is one of your primary duties because it influences how you coach and instruct your players and which strategies you might use during a game. So, know the rules, impart them to your players, and coach accordingly.

You can find more in-depth information on basketball rules on various websites and from youth basketball organizations.

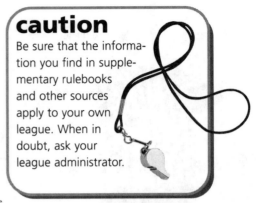

caution

Be sure that the information you find in supplementary rulebooks and other sources apply to your own league. When in doubt, ask your league administrator.

Teaching Rules to Your Players

To help your players know the rules, you need to know three things, in this order:

1. What your players *need* to know.
2. What they *do* know.
3. How to best impart what your players need to learn.

Your players need to know the basics: how to legally move the ball, what constitutes fouls and violations, what the consequences of those fouls and violations are, common terminology, and referee signals.

As you begin practicing and place your kids in game situations in practice, it will become evident which rules they know and which rules they don't know. At that point, it's up to you to make sure they learn what they need.

How should you go about teaching the rules to your players? Doing your best imitation of a classroom lecturer is definitely *not* the way to go. That will hold your players' attention for less than the time it takes to be called for a lane violation.

There are some effective ways you can teach the rules, though. Here are four ways you can help your players learn the rules of basketball:

- Situational plays
- Scrimmages
- Brief discussions
- Players' experiences

Let's take a look at each way.

Situational Plays

If you want your players to learn about screens, set up some plays to help them learn. Have players practice setting screens, brushing past screens, and defending against screens. Do the same for whatever skill or tactic you're working on: low-post play, fast breaks, perimeter ball movement, and so on.

The main point is to plan how to use your practice time and base your activities on what your players need to learn and improve on.

Scrimmages

You can also use scrimmages to see how much your players know and how they respond to various situations, and to teach them the correct response when they're unclear on what they should do. In this setting, your teaching focus is broader; you provide instruction in whatever area you see your players need it. In one moment, it might be on passing; a few minutes later it might be on dribble penetration; still later it might be on making the outlet pass on a fast break or learning how to effectively block out to rebound.

When you use scrimmages in this manner, you have a couple of choices: You can briefly stop play and instruct your players as the need arises, or you can note what you need to tell them and then discuss your point(s) at the end of practice. At times you'll find it necessary to stop the action to make your teaching point, or the moment will be lost. At other times, you can withhold the instruction for a break in the action, rather than disrupting the flow. In these latter cases, your point will be retained as well as if you had stopped the action to make it, and the flow of the action can go on uninterrupted.

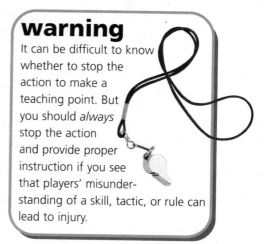

warning

It can be difficult to know whether to stop the action to make a teaching point. But you should *always* stop the action and provide proper instruction if you see that players' misunderstanding of a skill, tactic, or rule can lead to injury.

Brief Discussions

The end-of-practice discussion is also a good time to briefly teach or remind players of a rule (or anything else important) that they appeared to have difficulty understanding in that practice.

For example, you might say, "I noticed that sometimes we're camping in the lane too long. How long can you be in the lane before you have to move out?" Ideally, at least a few players will know the answer. If a player offers a correct answer, repeat it for everyone to hear. If no one responds correctly, tell them the answer and make a note to watch for fewer lane violations during the next practice.

Use these practice-ending discussions to briefly make a point, ideally a point that ties in directly to the activities of that practice. Don't drone on about various rules, especially if they don't relate to what the kids experienced that day. Kids learn better when the learning is practical and in context with what they're doing.

> **tip**
>
> Praising correct answers encourages responses to future questions. Never belittle players for incorrect answers. It makes them feel bad, and they will be less likely to participate in future team discussions.

Players' Experiences

Imagine the coach that teaches his players the rules by the book. He sits them down in orderly rows, lectures them for 50 minutes, and then gives them a written test, which they all ace. (I told you you'd have to use your imagination.)

> **note**
>
> In the next chapter you'll learn effective ways to communicate with your players, both during practice and in end-of-practice discussions.

Then the first game arrives, and the players have no idea what reaching in means, or why they can't change their pivot foot, or why they don't get to shoot every time they are fouled.

Book knowledge can't take the place of first-hand experience. Players learn the rules best when they see them applied in the practices and games they play in, especially when they are involved in the plays. *Then* the rules begin to register.

And that's good news because it means you don't have to spend your time lecturing to them about all the rules; you have to instruct along the way, as they play. And everyone—yourself included—has more fun that way.

Part of your job as coach is to reinforce your players' learning from practice to practice and game to game. As you observe their performances and discover what they need to learn, you can teach them not only the skills of basketball, but also the rules.

THE ABSOLUTE MINIMUM

This chapter focused on the basic rules of basketball—those pertaining to players, scoring, fouls, and violations. In addition, it provided terms you need to know, referees' signals, and ways to help your players learn. Keep in mind the following:

- You need to know not only the basic rules of basketball, but also any specific modifications your league has in place.

- Your players need to know the basic rules, and part of your responsibility is to determine what they do know and what they need to learn.

- After you know what your players need to learn, plan for effective ways to teach them the rules. These ways include using situational plays in practice, using scrimmages as teaching tools, holding brief end-of-practice discussions, and reinforcing players' learning through their own experiences gained through practices and games.

- You can expand your own knowledge of the rules by finding resources through your own league, through youth basketball organizations, and through resources you can find in your library or on the Web.

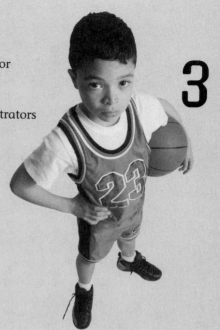

3

COMMUNICATĬON KEYS

As a coach, you're called on to do a lot of communicating. You address players, parents, other coaches, league administrators, and referees. You communicate in person, on the phone, in writing, one on one, and within group settings. How well you communicate with these groups significantly influences how successful your season is, how enjoyable it is, and how much your players learn.

Of course, you've been communicating all your life. It can't be that hard, right?

Right and wrong. If you haven't coached or taught before, and if you aren't used to instructing and leading youngsters, you are entering uncharted territory.

Consider this chapter your roadmap to help you chart that territory.

The 10 keys, presented first, will help you hone your communication skills as a coach. These keys are written with players in mind, but they apply to all groups with which you will communicate. Following the keys, we'll focus on the specifics of communicating with parents, league administrators, opponents, and referees.

10 Keys to Being a Good Communicator

Most people tend to think only of the verbal side of communication. That's important, but there's so much more to being a good communicator. Here are 10 keys to good communication:

1. Know your message.
2. Make sure you are understood.
3. Deliver your message in the proper context.
4. Use appropriate emotions and tones.
5. Adopt a healthy communication style.
6. Be receptive.
7. Provide helpful feedback.
8. Be a good nonverbal communicator.
9. Be consistent.
10. Be positive.

Know Your Message

Coach Caravelli gathers his players near a basket at the practice court and says, "All right, guys, today we're going to learn how to box out." He tells David to help him demonstrate, and asks Alex to put up a shot. Alex shoots, and as he does, Coach Caravelli spreads his legs and arms wide and sticks his rear out, trying to find David, but he keeps his eyes on the ball and the basket. David easily slips by him, untouched, and grabs the rebound.

"Just a lucky bounce," Coach mutters.

"But Coach, my dad says you're just supposed to find your man first, and then box out," one player says.

Coach Caravelli considers this a moment before saying, "Actually, let's just focus on shooting today. You guys like to shoot, right? Who wants to box out, anyway?"

The player was right; Coach Caravelli didn't know the technique for boxing out. He didn't really know his message.

Three issues are involved in knowing your message. You need to

- Know the skills and rules you need to teach.
- Read situations and respond appropriately.
- Provide accurate and clear information.

Know the Skills and Rules

Coach Caravelli didn't know how to teach the skill of boxing out. He might be a smooth, coherent, and clear speaker, but that's not going to help his players learn how to box out. Smoothness doesn't make up for lack of knowledge. You have to know the skills and rules.

> **tip**
>
> Coach Caravelli came to practice unprepared. Don't let that happen to you. Know what you're going to teach and how to teach it, including showing the proper technique. And if you don't know the proper technique, either shelve it for another practice so that you can learn the technique, or have your assistant coach or a skilled player demonstrate the technique.

Read the Situation

As Coach Caravelli teaches his players how to correctly execute screens, Kenny and Sam are quietly goofing off, not paying attention. But Coach Caravelli doesn't address the situation because they're not really disrupting his instruction and he's a little behind schedule. As his players begin to practice screens, Kenny and Sam are not executing as instructed. Kenny is not stationary when he sets screens, and Sam leaves a wide berth when running by the screener.

So Coach Caravelli stops the action and tells them how to properly execute screens. Then he lets them proceed.

Coach Caravelli delivered an important part of the message—Kenny and Sam need to know how to execute screens—but that was only part of the message he should have delivered. The real issue here was that the players weren't paying attention, and Coach Caravelli didn't correct the situation when it was occurring. He should have corrected that on the spot. Barring that, he should have told Kenny and Sam that the reason they didn't know how to execute a screen was because they weren't listening when he was teaching how to do so, and that they need to listen to his instruction the first time around.

> **caution**
>
> Eloquently stating and aptly showing how to perform a skill doesn't mean you're a good communicator if you can't keep your players' attention.

Sometimes knowing your message goes beyond understanding the content. You have to read the situation as well and tailor your message accordingly.

Provide Accurate and Clear Information

Knowing the content of your message isn't enough. You need to be able to deliver that content clearly and accurately.

Imagine a portion of a coach's preseason letter to parents reading like this:

> *"I'm really looking forward to coaching your child this season. Our first practice is next Monday at 6 p.m. See you then!"*

Too bad the coach didn't remember to note *where* the first practice is being held. As a result of not being clear in his letter, he'll have to spend a lot of time on the phone calling parents to deliver the information.

The same goes for teaching skills. Perhaps you know the proper technique for shooting, but your instruction is so technical and confusing that your players are worse off than if they had received no instruction at all! They're confused, you're frustrated, and no one learns how to shoot.

Know what information you need to deliver, and deliver it clearly so that all concerned understand. That's sometimes easier said than done.

Make Sure You Are Understood

As you can imagine, if you are not clear with your directives, you can create a lot of confusion. Take the following example:

> "Okay, Dion," Coach Hagan says, "the next time you're in that situation, make a crossover dribble and you'll shoot right past your defender. All right? Let's try it again."

Dion gives Coach Hagan a puzzled look, but Coach Hagan, in the midst of conducting a drill, doesn't notice. He's already getting the drill going again. Dion just hopes he's not in that same situation, because he has no idea what a crossover dribble is.

Just because something is clear to you doesn't mean it is clear to whomever you're delivering your message to, be it a player, a parent, an administrator, or anyone else. You need to watch for understanding and be ready to clarify your message if the person on the receiving end is confused.

When you state your message clearly and simply, you increase your chances of being understood. But don't count on that; instead, watch your players' facial expressions and read their body language. If they look confused or unsure of what to do, state your instruction again, making sure you use language they understand.

And watch how you say things: When you tell a player to "move to the vacated spot," she might not know that you mean to rotate to the open area that her teammate just left. Likewise, shouting out "Pick and roll! Pick and roll!" doesn't help if your players don't know what a pick and roll is.

Speak in language your players understand, and watch for their understanding.

Deliver Your Message in the Proper Context

In the first game of the season, Karim has just put up an awkward shot, using poor form. The ball is rebounded by the opponents, and a foul is called. As Karim moves downcourt before the ball is inbounded, Coach Grantham cups his hands to his mouth.

tip

A quizzical eye, a slumping shoulder, or a glazed look on a player's face speaks volumes. When you are able to understand your players' nonverbal communication, you are on the road to being a better communicator yourself.

"Hey, Karim! Use your fingers, not your palm! And square up your shoulders and hips to the basket! Remember to bend your knees to get a little momentum for your shot! And bend your shooting arm elbow to 45°. Don't forget to follow through!"

What's wrong with this? First, it's probably humiliating for Karim to have everyone in the gym witness his coach trying to instruct him on how to shoot. Second, it's not the time or place to give such detailed instruction. That should come in practice, not in games. The instruction itself wasn't incorrect; the timing of it was.

caution

Players' focus during games should be on the game itself, not on you giving them in-depth instruction.

Consider your context for delivering your message. Give brief reminders of tactical or skill execution during games, but save the teaching for practices.

Use Appropriate Emotions and Tones

Emotions are a natural part of basketball. Both you and your players (and their parents) can expect to experience a range of emotions throughout the season. In terms of communicating with others, your emotions can significantly affect your message.

How? Let's look at a few examples:

Situation: Devon, your point guard, is stationary, dribbling near the top of the key as his teammates are moving and cutting to get open. Jeff cuts toward the basket and is wide open for a moment. Devon is late with his pass, though, and the ball is knocked away and stolen.

Response #1: "Come on, Devon! Jeff was wide open! You can't fall asleep out there!"

Response #2: "That's all right! Let's get back on defense! Hold them, now. Let's get it back!"

Don't ever berate a player, publicly or privately. Remember that even National Basketball Association players make plenty of mistakes. Your players are going to make mistakes; what they need is instruction if they're not sure how to make a play, and encouragement, regardless. Help them to keep their focus on the game, not on how well they're pleasing you.

Situation: You are moments away from beginning the game that will decide your league championship.

Response #1: "All right, this is it, guys! There's no tomorrow. We've been playing to get to this game all year long. Show them what you're made of. I want to feel that championship trophy in my hands at the end of the game. How about you? Are you ready to go out and win?"

Response #2: "Okay, let's play basketball like we know how. Keep your focus on the fundamentals. Let's move the ball around, look for the open guy, play tough defense, and box out on the boards. Let's go have some fun, all right?"

Pep talks are better saved for the movies. Such talks often backfire because they get kids so sky high that they can't perform well. Your players need to focus on playing sound, fundamental basketball.

Situation: While practicing free throws, Terrell awkwardly slings the ball toward the basket, not using his legs at all.

Response #1: "Hey, Terrell, you look like you're shot-putting the ball up there! This isn't track and field, this is basketball!"

Response #2: "Use your legs, Terrell. Bend your knees to get a little momentum and strength. You can do it."

Sarcasm will get you nowhere. Terrell doesn't need sarcasm, or any type of humor. He needs instruction and encouragement.

Adopt a Healthy Communication Style

A lot of what you've been reading has to do with your communication style—whether you over-coach during games, offering too much instruction; whether you keep your emotions in check, or are too excitable or high-strung; what your tone is as you communicate; and so on. But there is more to consider concerning your communication style. It has to do with the bigger picture, with how you communicate on a daily basis. It has more to do with personality, outlook, and attitude than with reacting to a specific moment. And some styles are more effective than others.

Here are a few of the less-effective styles some coaches fall into:

- **Always talking, never listening**—Some coaches feel if they're not constantly talking, they're not providing the proper instruction their players need. Carried to the extreme, some feel that their players have nothing to say. Coaches who always talk and never listen tend to have players who stand around more in practice because their coach is talking, and those coaches don't get to know their players, thus missing out on one of the real joys of coaching basketball. *Deliver the messages you need to deliver, but don't feel you have to be talking throughout the entire practice.*

- **Always in control, too directive**—Some coaches run practices like drill sergeants, snapping orders at players, exerting their authority, and squelching fun wherever it begins to appear. When practice doesn't go exactly as they have choreographed it, they become irked. When players don't progress according to schedule, it drives them crazy. *Be in control of practice, yes, but don't squelch the fun and don't obsess over things you can't control.*

- **Not in control, too passive**—Other coaches take the opposite tack, either because they're unsure of themselves or they're too laid-back and give the impression that *no* one is in charge. They don't provide the guidance or discipline players need. Not comfortable in the spotlight, they avoid it, and discipline problems begin to crop up. *If you're a quiet or laid-back person, don't change your personality but do exert your authority as coach. You can be in charge and provide instruction without being loud and obnoxious.*

- **Seeking perfection**—There's a fine line between seeking to improve and seeking perfection. When coaches cross over the line into perfectionism, they are rarely satisfied with anything. Their forwards get rebounds, but their blocking out is not quite right. Shots go down, but there are flaws in the shooting mechanics. Even the gyms are not adequately lit or swept, at least in these coaches' eyes. Players are on edge when they play for a perfectionist coach; their focus turns from playing the game to pleasing the coach. *Help your players improve their skills, but allow them margin for mistakes. You can strive for improvement without putting added stress on the kids. Celebrate improvement even if it's still not picture-perfect.*

- **Not in control of emotions**—Some coaches throw up their hands in frustration when players are trying hard but having difficulty learning a skill. They shout in anger at a questionable call made by a volunteer referee. Their voices drip with sarcasm when players ask them something they feel the players should know. They respond with overzealous enthusiasm when their team scores a basket late in a game they are in control of, and this response is interpreted by all as unsporting behavior. *The point is not to suppress all your emotions, but to be in control of them. Consider the message you send with the* *emotion you show. Do suppress any urge to show your frustration toward kids who are trying to learn the skills, as well as any desire to express your anger on the court. Maintain your respect for the people involved in all situations. Your players need you to be steady and need to know what to expect from you.*

■ **Not aware of nonverbal communication**—Some coaches watch what they say but not what they do. They express their frustration or anger nonverbally, and if someone confronts them about that expression, they likely will say, "What? I didn't say anything." *Remember that you're communicating every second, whether verbally or nonverbally. Keep your nonverbal communication in line with your verbal communication, and make sure that both are positive, instructive, and encouraging.*

■ **Buddy-buddy with the players**—It's good to be friendly with players, but it's inappropriate to try to be their friend. Coaches who do this show a lack of maturity as they try to impress their players with how cool they are. *Have fun with your players, but maintain the coach-player relationship. You're there to help them become better ballplayers, not to become their pal.*

So, what *should* be your communication style?

You should provide the instruction your players need in a way that helps them improve their skills. To do this, you need good listening skills as well as good speaking skills, and you need to be encouraging and positive as you instruct and correct. Maintain respect for your players as you communicate with them. Be friendly and open with them, but don't try to become their friend. Create an enjoyable learning environment, maintain control over your emotions, and watch your nonverbal communication.

When you adopt this type of communication style, you're paving the way for your players to learn the game, improve their skills, and enjoy the season.

Be Receptive

A common mistake of new coaches is to assume that their sole role in communicating is to *talk*. Athletes are there to receive instruction, to be coached. Their focus should be on listening to you, on soaking in your instruction, on carrying out your commands.

There's plenty of truth in those statements, but they don't reflect the *whole* truth. Give your players room to speak, to ask questions, to voice opinions or concerns. In doing so, you can get to know them better and are

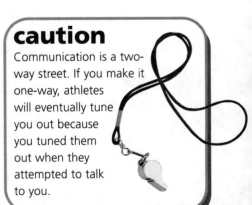

caution

Communication is a two-way street. If you make it one-way, athletes will eventually tune you out because you tuned them out when they attempted to talk to you.

better tuned in to their needs. Thus, you are more likely to pick up on issues and problems you need to deal with; see the following sidebar, "Dealing with Issues As They Arise."

Work at not only sending messages, but receiving them as well. As you talk to players, if you notice that their eyes are wandering or their bodies are turned partially away from you, they're sending you a message ("We're not really listening"). If their shoulders are slumped, their heads are down, or they're dragging their feet, they're sending one or more messages ("I'm tired"; "I'm discouraged"; "I'm bored"). If they're giving you a blank stare or have a dazed look, they're telling you they are tuning you out or are confused.

Don't ignore these signals. Handle them on a case-by-case basis. Each player will respond differently. Tune in, address the issues that need to be addressed, clarify instruction, and provide encouragement as needed, and keep your players on as even a keel as possible.

DEALING WITH ISSUES AS THEY ARISE

You might come across some discipline issues and other concerns you need to address as the season progresses. Here are some pointers on how to handle those issues:

- Let players know at the first practice how you expect them to behave, and let them know what the consequences of misbehavior will be. Write this down as well and give it to players or send it directly to their parents. This list needn't and shouldn't be long; it should be simple and clear and framed in a positive manner.

- Rather than just "laying down the law," consider involving your players in making team rules. Do this at the first practice. When they take part in making the rules and setting the consequences for breaking them, they might be more apt to stick to the rules. Giving players this type of responsibility promotes their emotional and social growth.

- When a player misbehaves, follow through as you had said you would.

- Don't tolerate razzing of teammates, taunting of opposing players, or other poor sporting behavior. Put a stop to such behavior, and follow through on any prescribed penalties.

- When a player needs extra help at practice in learning a skill, try to provide it on the spot, ideally using an assistant coach or a parent who volunteers to help. If the help can't be provided during that practice, other options might be to provide further instruction immediately following the practice or immediately preceding the next practice, in a one-on-one situation, if possible.

- When a player needs medical attention, provide the appropriate care immediately. You'll learn about this care in Chapter 4, "Safety Principles."

Provide Helpful Feedback

Tyler has been having trouble learning how to be a good defender. He tends to lunge for the ball, wanting to make a steal every time, and as a result he commits a lot of fouls. After one such foul, Tyler and his teammates return to the bench during a timeout.

> "Tyler, you need to stay on your man and play good defense," Coach Dixon says.

Is Coach Dixon telling Tyler something he doesn't already know? Hardly. Is he helping Tyler improve his defensive abilities? No. His feedback isn't helpful at all; if anything, it just adds to the pressure Tyler undoubtedly already feels.

Coach Dixon should focus on giving specific, practical feedback that will help Tyler improve his defense. You'll learn about this type of feedback in Chapter 6, "Player Development." For now, know that such feedback is one of your duties in communicating with your players, and when it's given properly, it can reap great dividends in terms of player improvement.

Be a Good Nonverbal Communicator

Studies have shown that up to 70% of communication is accomplished nonverbally. You just read about the importance of reading nonverbal cues—watching facial expressions and body language. You also have to pay attention to the nonverbal cues you send:

> "Way to go, Alex!" Coach Dintiman says, clapping his hands and smiling.
>
> "Way to go, Alex!" Coach Garner says, arms crossed tightly across his chest and a scowl on his face.

The same words were used, but Coach Garner sent a vastly different message than Coach Dintiman.

Nonverbal messages are being sent constantly—both with and without words. Consider your facial expressions during practices and games. Sometimes it's appropriate to show that you're frustrated—for example, when kids are goofing off. But when kids are exerting themselves on the court and not executing well, keep your frustration in check. Consider what messages your expressions and body language are sending, and make sure those messages are what you *want* to be sending.

Be Consistent

Your players need consistency from you in three ways. They need consistency

- In the messages you send
- In how you treat them
- In your temperament and style

Consistent Messages

If you hear different messages from the same person on the same topic, what happens? You begin not to trust that person. The same happens if one week your players hear you say, "We're hurrying our shots! I want to see at least three passes each time before we put up a shot," only to hear you follow that the next week with, "Terry, you were wide open for that shot! You've got to take that opportunity when you get it!" (This latter advice came after Terry received the first pass and was dutifully looking to pass.)

> # caution
> Remember, if your body language conflicts with your words, players will be just as confused as if you told them one thing one day, and the opposite thing the next. Keep your body language in line with the verbal messages you send.

Confusing? You bet. If you do this often, the players will not know what to believe, no matter what you say. Be sure you send consistent messages.

Consistent Treatment

Make sure you treat all your players in similar fashion. If Dan breaks a team rule one week and you discipline him accordingly, and the next week Zach breaks the same rule but you overlook it because he's one of your best players, what message does that send to your team? That it's okay to break the rules if you're good enough?

Likewise, if you spend more of your time with your average and good players in hopes of turning them into good and great players, respectively, what does that say to the lesser-skilled players? That they don't matter because they can't shoot or defend as well as their teammates?

All your players need your attention and guidance to improve. They need to adhere to the same team rules and be treated the same way if they break those rules. And they all need to know that they are equally valued by you, regardless of their playing abilities.

> # tip
> So how do you fairly penalize a starter and a substitute for the same infraction? One approach is to take an equal amount of playing time from them both—say, five minutes. Start the starter, but take five minutes from his time.
>
> The main point is to think through your penalties and assess them as evenly as possible.

Know that after your season starts and you name your starters, players (and parents) will feel that the substitutes are not quite as valued as the starters. At the younger levels, you might rotate starting responsibilities from game to game and thus avoid this dilemma, but at older levels, you'll be starting your best players.

So how do you handle this? First, make sure you give equal attention and help to all your players in practice. They not only deserve this attention, but they need it to contribute in their substitute roles. It helps your team when *everyone* improves, not just your starters.

Second, let players know how the middle and end of the game is just as important as the beginning. If you have 5 or 10 or 15 minutes to play, no matter what segments of the game those minutes come in, the team needs every player to contribute.

Third, emphasize that not everyone is going to be a scoring machine, and reward players for all the other things—big and small—that contribute to wins: rebounds, tough defense, steals, assists, and so on. Find ways to tangibly reward substitutes who play well, doing the "little things" that often go unnoticed. Don't let them go unnoticed on your team!

Consistent Style

They also need to know what to expect from you. If you are patient and encouraging one practice and moody or volatile the next, the learning environment suffers (as do the players). We all have mood swings, and we're not robots. But do strive to be even-keeled and consistent in your approach from practice to practice, setting aside any personal issues that might affect your mood and your communication with your players on any given day.

Be Positive

Kids learn best in a positive environment. Give them sound instruction, consistent encouragement, and plenty of understanding. Note, however, that being positive doesn't mean letting kids run all over you, and it doesn't mean having a Pollyanna attitude where you falsely praise a player for almost getting a rebound if, by using good technique, she should have easily gotten the rebound. It means you instruct and guide your players as they learn and practice skills and give them the sincere encouragement and praise they need as they work to hone their abilities. You'll learn more about how to use praise in Chapter 6.

note

These 10 keys not only apply to how you communicate with your players, but should also guide your communication with parents, referees, other coaches, and administrators.

Communicating with Parents

Although most communication happens between coaches and players, important communication takes place between coaches and parents, too. In this section, we'll consider the various times and ways you should communicate with parents and learn how to handle challenging situations and involve parents in positive ways throughout the season.

Preseason Meeting or Letter

You'll need to contact parents before the season begins. You can communicate the following information at a parents' meeting or through a letter. If you hold a parents' meeting, it's still helpful to give parents a handout that covers the items you talk about, so they can have written information to refer to later. In your preseason meeting or letter, consider including the following items:

- **Introduction**—Tell parents who you are, what your coaching background is (if you have one), and how you got involved coaching the team. Make this brief, but know that parents appreciate knowing a bit about who will be coaching their sons and daughters.

- **Your coaching philosophy**—Let parents know your approach to coaching, including your philosophy in terms of providing instruction, giving all players equal playing time, and so on. Tell them, briefly, *why* this is your philosophy and how it benefits the kids.

- **The inherent risks**—Basketball has some inherent risks you need to make parents aware of. You should also let them know you have a plan in place to respond to injuries, and find out from parents any medical conditions their children have, as well as how the parents can be contacted in case of an emergency. You'll learn more about this in Chapter 4.

- **Basic expectations**—State your expectations of players and parents in a positive fashion, and let parents know what they and their children can expect of you as a coach.

- **The practice schedule**—Include the day, date, time, and place of the first practice, and note the rest of the practice schedule if you know it at this time.

- **The game schedule**—If you know the game schedule, include that as well. If not, let parents know when they can expect to receive the schedule.

- **Other information**—If you have some special event planned or want to invite parents to volunteer to help in various ways, inform parents in your meeting or letter.

- **Your contact information**—Let parents know how and when they can contact you.

For a sample preseason letter, see Appendix A, "Sample Letter to Parents."

Preseason Call

Even with a preseason letter or meeting, it's wise to call parents of players before the first practice to remind them of the time and place of that practice. Otherwise, you'll likely have players who don't show up for the first practice.

During the Season

After the season is underway, you'll have numerous opportunities to communicate with parents: as kids are being dropped off or picked up at practice, after games, and on the phone or through email at other times of the week. Here are some pointers on doing so:

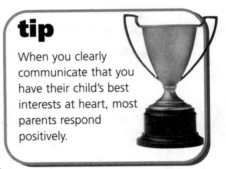

tip

When you clearly communicate that you have their child's best interests at heart, most parents respond positively.

- If you have a few minutes immediately before or after practice, that's a good time to meet parents, get to know them a little bit, match faces with names, and enlist help if you need it. It's also a good time to let parents know what they can do to help their child. For example, you could suggest to Ramon's parents that if they had time, they could work with him at home on dribbling with his left hand, or you could let Tara's parents know she could use some practice making crisper passes. Parents like to know what they can do to help their son or daughter.

- Ask parents to let you know when their child is not going to be at a game. Also let them know they can talk with you about any concerns they have about their child.

- Let parents know what type of communication is allowed during games. Whatever boundaries you set here, do so with the players in mind and what will help them focus on the game the most. Most coaches prefer not to have any direct parental intervention during a game, meaning shouting encouragement from the stands is fine, but going to the bench to talk to their child is not. Some coaches don't mind parents coming by the bench and chatting briefly with the players; this is up to you. Just let parents know what your preferences are here, and ask that they respect them.

- Likewise, let parents know what's appropriate immediately after games. Many coaches like to spend five minutes or so talking to their players, reinforcing what went well and talking about what they still need to work on. At younger ages, post-game sometimes means snack time as well. Whatever your protocol, let parents know, and let them know if and how they can be appropriately involved.

■ Scheduling changes call for communicating with parents, too. If a game or practice is rescheduled, you can contact parents in whatever way you've set up: by yourself, with the aid of an assistant coach, or by phone tree. (A *phone tree* is a system that links all families together. For example, on a team of 10 players, you could have 2 or 3 parents—the "branches"—help you make the calls, rather than you calling all 12 families. You should have set up this tree beforehand.)

Whichever way you decide, though, make sure parents are contacted by phone when a practice or game is rescheduled. Even if parents say email is a good way to contact them, chances are that not all parents will check their email in time.

Be Understanding—and Set Boundaries

Most parents are there to cheer on their kids. Parents want to see their kids do their best, have fun, and succeed. It's thrilling for a parent to watch her child score a basket or make a great steal. And it's painful for a parent to watch her son dribble the ball off his foot or see her daughter miss a shot in a crucial situation. It's likely that parents experience more emotional highs and lows watching their children play than do the players and coaches who are directly involved in the game.

You need to understand the experience from the parents' point of view and create an environment that allows parents to be positively involved throughout the season. Indeed, you should encourage such participation. (For suggestions on how to do this, see the sidebar "Involving Parents.")

At the same time, you need to set boundaries for parents and be prepared to handle situations that can detract from the players' experience. Some of those situations and boundaries are addressed in the "Challenging Situations" section.

INVOLVING PARENTS

Some parents present challenges to coaches. But most want to support the team and its coach. Help parents know how they can be involved with your team in positive ways. Here are a few ideas:

■ **Encourage support**—Ask parents to be positive and vocal in their support of each player and to display good sporting behavior. Their main role at games is to cheer on their team.

■ **Ask for help**—If you don't have an assistant coach, ask if any parent would like to volunteer. Even if you do have an assistant, having parents volunteer to help at practice can be beneficial because you can break the players into smaller units and thus give them more touches of the ball. Also, you might want to set up parents on a snack schedule, with a different parent or set of parents responsible for providing a team snack at each game. You also might set up a phone tree with parents, as mentioned earlier, so important information can be quickly passed on.

In addition, if you and your assistant coach don't like to keep a scorebook, you might find that a parent wouldn't mind that task.

■ **Build camaraderie**—Social gatherings are nice ways to build camaraderie among parents and team family members. Consider having a midseason potluck or pizza party to help families get to know each other better, or plan other social events that foster open communication and deepened relationships. And parents are often more than willing to step to the fore and organize such events—so let them!

Challenging Situations

You might not have any challenging situations with parents. But it's best to be prepared for those challenges and know how to respond, just in case. Following are some of the challenges coaches can face and suggestions for how to handle them.

Parents Who Coach from the Bleachers

At some time during the season, you might experience the following:

> "Work the give and go! You need to run the give and go!" one parent yells early in the game. "Send Marcy in! She could stop that hot shot!" another yells a little later. "Get the ball in to Jason down low!" instructs a third parent.

It's one thing to encourage players from the bleachers; it's quite another to coach them from that vantage point. It's not a matter of whether the instruction is good; it's a matter of where that instruction is coming from. Coaching advice is your domain.

If you hear parents of your players coaching from the bleachers, remind your players to focus on what you say, not on what they hear elsewhere. Then, after the game, talk to the parents who were coaching from the bleachers. Tell them they need to focus their support on cheering on the team, not on telling them how to play. It's confusing and disconcerting for players to hear instruction from the bleachers, even if it's in line with what you've told them. And quite often that instruction flies in the face of what you've told them.

In any case, coaching from the bleachers is disruptive and inappropriate. Tell the offending parents this and request that they refrain from it in the future.

Parents Who Demand That You Coach Their Child Differently

There is also the possibility you will have parents who just don't think you are doing a good job with their child. Take some of the following sample comments:

> "My kid should be the starting point guard in our playoff game, not Derrick. If you want to win that game, you should be starting my kid."

"What's the deal with giving everyone all this playing time? My kid's the best player on the team, and he shouldn't be sitting out at all, unless it's a blowout."

"Why don't you play Tyler more than Jeremy? Tyler has a much better shot, and he's quicker, too. Tyler should be playing a lot more, if you ask me."

Well, you *didn't* ask that parent, and you didn't ask the other parents for their "advice," either. But sometimes you get it, free of charge.

Don't get into a long conversation with parents on how you coach their child. You don't need to defend your right to make coaching decisions. Tell parents politely and firmly that while you appreciate their concerns, those are coaching decisions reserved for you and any assistant coaches you might have. Remind them that the decisions you make are in the best interest of all the players, including their own son or daughter. And leave it at that.

Parents Who Yell at Referees

If you've attended many youth basketball games, you've probably heard comments like the following:

"C'mon, ref! That was a foul!"

"Hey, ref! Want to borrow my glasses?"

"That's terrible! He calls the ticky-tack fouls, but not the obvious ones!"

Are parents justified in making derogatory or disparaging comments to or about referees? Absolutely not, even if the referee misses the call. Youth league referees are most often volunteers, unpaid and untrained. Yelling at the referee is poor sporting behavior, and it sends the wrong message to kids:

If I was called for a foul, it was because the referee doesn't know basketball. If we lost, it was because of lousy refereeing.

It tells kids it's okay to disrespect the referee, it takes their focus off their own performances, and it implies that the game's outcome is far more important than it really is. It also usurps part of your role, which is to calmly discuss with referees certain calls (these debates should be rare; you'll learn more about them in "Communicating with Opponents and Referees" later in this chapter).

As noted earlier, let parents know up front what you expect of them, including their behavior at games. If they yell at the referees during games, talk with them after the game. Perhaps call them a little later in the evening, after they've had time to cool off. Tell them you appreciate their support but that you need them to stop berating the referees, even if they miss calls. Tell them why you feel this way (for the reasons stated in the previous paragraph), and ask that they refrain from doing so at future games.

Parents Who Yell at Their Own Kids

Parents who yell at their own kids—for missing shots, for making bad passes, for whatever reason—do a tremendous disservice to their children. The words of parents are extremely powerful, and they have the power to damage and destroy. Sadly, sports seem to be an arena in which some parents choose to harm their children's egos. Those damaging words reverberate in the youngster's ears long past the game and far from the court.

If a parent yells at his child during a game, counter the harmful words with your own words of encouragement and sincere praise. Just make sure the praise is truly sincere because kids can see through false praise and such praise can undermine your own credibility and their ability to believe you in this or other situations.

If you believe the situation warrants it, talk to that parent during the game or send a nonverbal message to him to cut the negative talk. Before doing this, though, consider whether you can send your message without fanning the flames on the spot. You don't want an escalated confrontation; you want the parent to stop yelling at his kid.

If you don't communicate with the parent on the spot, do so after the game, one on one. Tell the parent that his son needs his support and encouragement. If he can't provide that support and encouragement, ask the parent to stop attending games.

Parents Who Yell at Other Kids

Many parents cheer on their own kids but loudly disparage other players, either on their own child's team or on the opposing team. Take the following examples:

> "Hey, this kid can't handle the ball! He's going to get it stolen!"

> "Come on, you should've gotten that rebound!"

> "Hey, nice pass!" (A comment made with dripping sarcasm.)

Don't tolerate this any more than you would tolerate parents verbally abusing their own child. Intervene in the same way you would with a parent yelling at her own son or daughter.

Parents Who Abuse Their Children

Children can be abused physically, emotionally, and sexually. The signs of abuse are not always readily apparent, nor are they always easily separated from the scratches and bruises that come from normal childhood activity.

The point here is not to make you paranoid and suspect abuse when you see a player with a black eye, but to keep your own eyes open and watch for additional signs. Kids who are abused tend to

■ Have a poor self-image

■ Act out in practice or at games

- Be withdrawn, passive, or sad
- Lash out angrily at their peers
- Bully or intimidate weaker peers
- Have difficulty trusting others
- Be self-disparaging or self-destructive

Players who exhibit some or all of these signs might have been abused, or they might have experienced another child being abused. Complicating matters, these signs are also exhibited by kids who are undergoing various types of stress—for example, their parents' recent divorce.

If you do suspect that one of your players is being abused, it's your responsibility to contact the proper authorities— your local child protection services agency, police, hospital, or an emergency hotline. In many cases, you can do so anonymously. In any regard, if you have reason to believe abuse might be taking place, report it.

> **note**
>
> What you're trying to do in all these situations is turn a win-lose situation into a win-win situation. You don't want to defeat parents; you want to win them over so that you're on the same side, with the end result being that the players benefit.

Communicating with League Administrators

Part of a league administrator's role is to set up and administer leagues. Administrators schedule games, set up league policies and rules, oversee the maintenance of the courts, dispense the necessary equipment, arrange for officiating, and take care of many other responsibilities, all with the goal of providing a top-quality experience for the players.

A coach's interaction with league administrators generally falls into three categories:

- League information
- Coaches' meetings and clinics
- Questions and concerns

Let's look at each of these in the following sections.

League Information

The league should provide information on game schedules, practice court usage, equipment distribution, league policies and rules, and any upcoming coaches' meetings or clinics. Read the information you receive; make copies of the game schedules for parents; and talk with your administrator if you have any questions about the schedule, the policies, or any other information dispensed by the league.

Coaches' Meetings and Clinics

Most leagues hold a preseason coaches' meeting at which the administrator distributes the necessary information and updates coaches on new policies, modified rules, and other important matters.

Some leagues also conduct coaches' training. If your league offers such training, take advantage of it.

The point here is to consider ways to help you better prepare for your season. Coaching clinics and courses are one good way to do so.

> **tip**
>
> The American Sport Education Program (www.asep.com) offers effective training courses for youth coaches, including an online course in youth basketball. This is one of many good programs that can be found.

Questions and Concerns

Take any overarching questions or concerns—about league policies or rules, practice court availability, scheduling, and so on—to your league administrator. In addition, if you have an ongoing problem with a parent and are unable to resolve it with that parent, consider talking with your league administrator. By all means, do so if the problem affects the enjoyment of the game for other fans, the parent poses some sort of physical threat to anyone, or the parent is verbally abusive at games and refuses to stop or leave when she becomes abusive.

Communicating with Opponents and Referees

Three key words here: *respect*, *dignity*, *restraint*.

Besides being your players' coach, you are also their role model, whether you like it or not. And how you communicate with opposing coaches, players, and referees speaks volumes about what kind of role model you are.

If you have a question for a referee, ask it at the proper time and without showing up the referee or unnecessarily slowing the game. Treat the referees and the opposing coaches with the same respect you'd like to be shown.

At the ends of games, line up your players and lead them as you shake hands with the other

> **note**
>
> You can teach your kids all the requisite skills, but if you don't teach them how to play the game—all-out, having fun, and showing respect for the referees and opponents—you haven't taught them enough.

team. Instruct your players to be respectful as they shake or slap hands. Also thank the referees for volunteering their time.

THE ABSOLUTE MINIMUM

This chapter was all about what, when, and how to communicate with your players, parents, league administrators, opposing coaches and players, and referees. Key points included

- Use the 10 keys to being a good communicator. Those keys are 1) Know your message; 2) Make sure you are understood; 3) Deliver your message in the proper context; 4) Use appropriate emotions and tones; 5) Adopt a healthy communication style; 6) Be receptive; 7) Provide helpful feedback; 8) Be a good nonverbal communicator; 9) Be consistent; and 10) Be positive.

- Contact parents before the season begins, sharing information about your coaching philosophy and practice and game schedules, and paving the way for healthy communication throughout the season.

- Let parents know what you expect of them in terms of positive team support, and what they can expect of you.

- Suggest ways parents can be actively involved in supporting and helping the team.

- Work through the challenging situations parents sometimes present. Keep your players' best interests in mind as you work for win-win situations.

- If you have reason to believe a player has been abused, report it to local authorities.

- Give the referees and opponents the same respect you would like to be shown. Be a model of good sporting behavior for your players.

- Communicating the inherent risks
- Being prepared
- Providing proper supervision
- Responding to minor injuries
- Responding to emergency situations

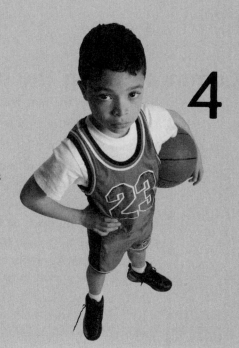

4

SAFETY PRINCIPLES

Basketball is a contact sport. Bodies collide, fouls occur, and kids fall down. Injuries do occur at the youth level.

Sometimes those injuries are preventable, and sometimes they aren't. This chapter focuses on how to create a safe environment for your players, provide the supervision they need, and do all you can to prevent injuries. You'll also learn how to respond to the injuries that do happen. Hopefully you won't have an emergency to respond to, but if you do, you need to know what action to take, so you'll learn about that as well.

Communicating the Inherent Risks

A player drives the lane and two defenders converge on him.

Three players battle for a rebound under the basket.

Two players dive for a loose ball near the sideline.

A player sets a screen on a defender who doesn't see the screener.

These are just some of the situations that can lead to injuries in basketball. Most of the injuries are along the lines of scrapes, bruises, jammed fingers, and twisted ankles. Major injuries are rare, but they can occur.

Like all sports, basketball has its inherent risks. It's your duty to communicate these risks to parents. As mentioned in Chapter 3, "Communication Keys," you should do this before the season starts, either in a letter or in a parent meeting.

What should you say? Tell the parents about the types of injuries that can occur. Assure them that you will do all in your power to prevent injuries, but that you can't prevent all injuries, and parents and players should understand the risks going in.

Ask parents to equip their children with shoes that provide support and traction. Let parents know you will do your part in providing adequate supervision at practices and games.

Many leagues have consent forms parents must fill out. In doing so, parents acknowledge that they understand the risks involved and do not hold the coach or the league liable for injuries that occur while players are participating in the program.

warning

Consent forms do not protect you from all liability issues. If you do not provide adequate supervision or respond appropriately to an injured player, you can still be held liable. However, by being able to prove that you provided proper supervision and instruction, you are less likely to be held accountable for a player's injury.

Being Prepared

There are several actions you can take to be prepared to handle injury and emergency situations. Three of those actions include

- Having CPR/first aid training
- Being prepared to respond to kids with chronic health conditions
- Having a well-stocked first aid kit on hand

Beyond these, you should also have a plan for responding to both minor injuries and major injuries. You'll learn more about those plans a little later in this chapter. For now, let's take a look at the three items just mentioned.

CPR/First Aid Training

CPR and first aid training is often offered through local hospitals and medical clinics, as well as through national organizations such as the American Red Cross. Sports leagues often sponsor or arrange for the training, which covers the basics of providing cardiopulmonary resuscitation and first aid for a variety of injuries.

If you have the opportunity to be trained in CPR/first aid, take it. Understanding the proper response and practicing the correct techniques involved go much further than reading about the topic.

If you don't have the opportunity to be trained, study this chapter carefully and supplement your learning with additional resources as you see fit.

Chronic Health Condition Awareness

Dontrelle races hard downcourt on a fast break and is thankful when the whistle blows and a foul is called. He bends over and puts his hands on his knees, wheezing hard; he can't seem to catch his breath. His wheezing is beyond the normal out-of-breath, out-of-shape gasping for air. He is truly having trouble getting enough air into his lungs. What do you do?

Right before she got to the gym, Hannah was stung by a bee. Inside the gym, her eyes begin to itch and swell. She develops hives and begins wheezing. How do you respond?

Tyler begins sweating and trembling. He is turning pale. You know he is diabetic. What action do you take?

Dontrelle has asthma, Hannah is allergic to bee stings, and Tyler (as mentioned) suffers from diabetes. These are examples of chronic conditions that some of your players might have and that you might have to deal with as your season progresses. With chronic health conditions, it's vital that you

- Are aware that the child has the condition
- Know the signs the child will exhibit when the condition is bothering him
- Know how to respond to the symptoms

Before the first practice, have parents fill out a medical emergency form (see Appendix B, "Medical Emergency Form"). On this form they can note what type of allergy or condition their children have, which symptoms to watch for, what to do in case of an attack or episode, and at what phone numbers they can be reached.

If parents note an allergy or condition but are sparse with their information on what signs to look for, ask them directly what you should watch for. You can also find this information easily on the Internet or through resources in your library.

Just as important as knowing what to look for is knowing how to respond. The child's parents are the first and most important resource here; they will know what treatment is called for. Some situations will call for you to seek immediate emergency help. Know what these situations are and carry the appropriate medical emergency numbers—and a cell phone, if possible—with you at practices and games. If you don't have a cell phone, carry change with you for a pay phone.

First Aid Kit

Stock a first aid kit and take it with you to practices and games. Some stores sell complete kits; you can buy an already-assembled kit or put one together on your own. Either way, here are the essentials you should have on hand:

- Phone numbers of parents, players' doctors, emergency medical personnel, and police
- Change for a pay phone
- Antiseptic wipes
- Antibacterial soap
- First aid cream
- Instant cold pack
- Gauze rolls
- Triangular bandages
- 2" elastic bandage
- Bandages, sheer and flexible, of various sizes
- Nonstick pads of assorted sizes
- Hypoallergenic first aid tape
- Oval eye pads
- Acetaminophen
- Scissors
- Tweezers
- Insect sting kit
- Disposable gloves
- First aid guide
- Contents card

tip

Use the contents card to remind you of what you *should* have and what you *do* have, so you know when to restock. Use the first aid guide to help you remember how to care for minor injuries (it's easier than carrying this book with you to practice).

Providing Proper Supervision

In the rush to provide superior coaching and teaching and to shape their youngsters into the best possible basketball players over the course of a season, many coaches overlook an even more important duty—to provide proper supervision at practices and games.

Parents are entrusting their children to you; your most important duty is to make sure their kids are cared for and supervised in a safe environment.

To provide the supervision your players need, be sure you

- Plan your practices.
- Inspect the court and equipment.
- Provide proper instruction.
- Supervise each activity.

Plan Your Practices

In Chapter 5, "Practice Plans," you'll learn how to plan your season and individual practices. Planning prepares you to instruct and coach more effectively. When you're organized, know what you want to teach, and know how you want to teach it, you're more likely to stay on task and maintain control. In turn, your players are more likely to stay focused, taking their cues from you, and less likely to have down time to fool around while you're figuring out what to do next.

You'll learn to plan your practices using a logical progression of skills, based on your players' level of development and physical condition.

Keep these season and practice plans; they can be important if an injury were to occur and your judgment in terms of planning were questioned. Also fill out and keep any injury reports (see Appendix C, "Injury Report") for your records.

Inspect the Court and Equipment

Check your practice and game courts before playing on them. Look for water or slippery areas, for chipped or broken tiles or boards, and any conditions that might lead to injury. Report these conditions to your league administrator.

Provide Proper Instruction

If your players don't know the fundamentals of rebounding, of driving to the hoop, of screening, and of many other aspects of the game, they put themselves and others at risk. That's why it's so important that you teach your players the proper technique for all the skills they need to perform. It not only increases their chances of playing well, but also decreases their chances of being injured.

Supervise Each Activity

Planning the practice, knowing what you want your players to be doing from minute to minute, isn't enough. You need to closely supervise the players as they participate in each activity. Accidents and injuries are more likely to happen when activities are not supervised.

That means don't get kids started in an activity and then watch them out of the corner of your eye while you make a call on your cell phone. It also means not temporarily leaving the court, entrusting the players to the charge of your teenage son. It means staying focused on the activity, being there to provide feedback on players' performances, and—most importantly from a legal standpoint—ensuring that the activity is conducted safely and that all players are under your direct supervision.

tip

Two more safety tips: One, stretch and warm up properly for practices and games. And two, remember that your players are kids, not miniature adults. Their bodies can't take the physical stress that adults' bodies can. Don't encourage kids to play through pain, and don't expect them to do what you can do.

Responding to Minor Injuries

The focus so far has been on doing all you can to prevent injuries from occurring. Still, they will occur, and you need to know how to respond to them.

Most of the injuries in youth basketball are minor: scrapes and bruises, sprains and strains. Here's how you should respond in each situation.

Cuts and Scrapes

Remember the disposable gloves in your first aid kit? Here's where you use them—as a barrier between you and a player's blood. While wearing the gloves, stop the bleeding by pressing directly on the cut with a gauze bandage. If the cut is deep enough that blood soaks the bandage, keep that bandage in place and apply another one.

When the bleeding has stopped, remove the gauze bandage and cleanse the wound with an antiseptic wipe. Apply some first aid cream. Then place a clean bandage over the wound.

tip

A player with a bloody nose should lean slightly forward and pinch shut his nostrils. The bleeding should stop within several minutes. If it doesn't, seek medical help.

Bruises

Things sometimes go bump in the night. More often, they go bump under the basket, or on a fast break, or during a screen. Wherever the bump takes place, a bruise often results. Many bruises don't need any special treatment, but if the area is swollen and tender, treat it through the PRICE method:

- **P = Protect**—Keep the athlete from further harm as you tend to the injury.
- **R = Rest**—This hastens the healing process.
- **I = Ice**—This reduces inflammation in the injured area, which aids in the healing process; it also reduces the pain.
- **C = Compress**—When you compress the injured area with a tightly secured ice bag (use an elastic bandage to do this), you ensure that the ice can do its job.
- **E = Elevate**—When you raise the injured area above the heart level, this minimizes the amount of blood that pools in the area. The more blood that pools in the area, the longer the injury will take to heal.

tip

Apply ice for about 15 minutes every 3 hours or so during the day. When the swelling decreases, the player can begin gentle range-of-motion exercises for the affected joint.

Sprains and Strains

A *sprain* happens when ligaments or tendons are stretched too far from their normal position. Typically, a sprain occurs in the ankle, knee, or wrist. A sprain generally causes pain, swelling, and bruising of the affected joint.

A *strain* occurs when a muscle is stretched too far. In basketball, the most common strains are to hamstrings (the muscles in the backs of the thighs).

Treat sprains and strains with the PRICE method. The player should fully recover and gradually work back to full speed.

Remember to use the injury report to keep a record of all injuries, including minor ones.

note

Overuse injuries result from the stress placed on bodies by repetitive training. Such injuries can include stress fractures, strains, sprains, tendonitis, bursitis, and shin splints.

RETURNING AFTER AN INJURY

Most players want to return from an injury as soon as possible. But if they return too quickly, they can aggravate the injury and end up missing more action than necessary.

Here are some guidelines for when injured players can return to action:

■ They should return when they have been cleared to do so by their parents and, if appropriate, by their doctor.

■ They should not practice or play if they still feel pain in the injured area during rest.

■ They should use simple exercises to gently work the injured area after they have no pain at rest.

■ If they feel pain as they resume exercising, they should stop.

■ They should return gradually to full intensity, listening to their bodies and increasing intensity only when they can do so without pain.

Responding to Emergency Situations

You need to be prepared to respond to emergency situations, such as broken bones and head, neck, and back injuries. An emergency situation can also crop up with a chronic health condition. Your role here is not to treat the player, but to facilitate that treatment while protecting the player from further harm.

To do so, you need to have an emergency plan in place. Here are the essentials of such a plan:

1. Evaluate the player and use your CPR/first aid training as appropriate. However, do *not* move, or allow the movement of, a player who has suffered a neck or back injury, a dislocated joint, or a broken bone.

2. Contact medical personnel, reassure the child, keep others away from him, and remain with the child until medical help arrives. Assign an assistant coach or a parent to call medical personnel, if possible. It's ideal that you stay with the player, to keep her calm.

3. If the child is taken to the hospital and her parents are not available to go with her, appoint an assistant coach or a parent to accompany the child. Ideally, this person will be someone the player knows and can take comfort from.

tip

Always carry these phone numbers with you at practices and games: players' parents (home, office, and mobile phones), players' physicians, hospital, police, and rescue unit. Also be sure you have players' emergency information on hand. You'll gain this information through the form found in Appendix B.

Heatstroke

In heatstroke, a person's body temperature climbs dangerously high as heat is generated more quickly than the body can handle it. As the body's thermoregulatory mechanisms fail, heatstroke can occur. In the late stages of heatstroke, the person loses his ability to sweat, but this isn't the case earlier on.

Signs of heatstroke include

- Fatigue and weakness
- Nausea and vomiting
- Headache
- Dizziness
- Muscle cramps
- Irritability

A person suffering from heatstroke has hot, flushed skin. He likely also has a rapid pulse, shallow breathing, and constricted pupils. The person might exhibit strange behavior and confusion.

What should you do if a player exhibits some of these signs? If you're outside, get the player into shade. Have him sit or lie down, remove any excess clothing or equipment, and cool his body with wet towels or by pouring cold water over him. Have someone call medical personnel immediately. Have the player drink cool water. Another way to cool the body is to place ice packs on the armpits, neck, and back and between the legs.

Under no circumstances should you allow an athlete who has suffered heatstroke to return to action until he has been examined by a doctor and cleared to play.

Heat Exhaustion

Heat exhaustion happens when a person becomes dehydrated. This person usually is sweating profusely and has pale, clammy skin; a rapid and weak pulse; dilated pupils; and a loss of coordination.

The signs of heat exhaustion are the same as for heatstroke. The treatment is also the same, with the exception that you might not need to send for medical personnel. Send for medical personnel if the player's condition doesn't improve or if it worsens. Again, don't let the player resume practicing or playing without the consent of her physician.

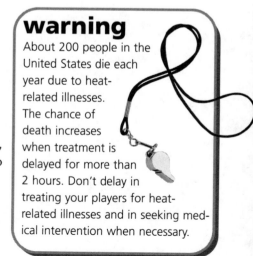

warning

About 200 people in the United States die each year due to heat-related illnesses. The chance of death increases when treatment is delayed for more than 2 hours. Don't delay in treating your players for heat-related illnesses and in seeking medical intervention when necessary.

THE ABSOLUTE MINIMUM

This chapter is intended to prepare you to provide for the safety of your players. Among the main points are these:

- Let parents know of the inherent risks of playing basketball before the season begins.

- There are many ways you can prepare yourself to provide for safety. Among them are being trained in CPR/first aid, being aware of any chronic health conditions of your players, knowing how to respond if a player's health condition flares up, and having a well-stocked first aid kit on hand at all practices and games.

- One of your most important duties is to provide proper supervision at practices and games. This comes through planning your practices, inspecting the court and equipment, providing proper instruction, and closely supervising each activity.

- Know how to respond to minor injuries, including cuts and scrapes, bruises, and sprains and strains.

- Have an emergency plan in place, have all the important phone numbers you need in case of an emergency, and enact the plan when a major injury happens.

5

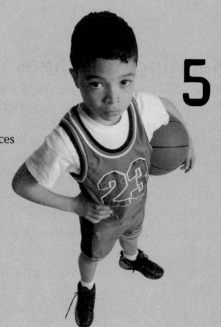

PRACTICE PLANS

Generally, the people who volunteer their time—such as for coaching—are already busy people. Now they add one more thing to their plate. And then, in the few quiet moments of their day (usually lasting no more than 30 seconds), they wonder how they are going to find the time to fulfill their latest volunteer obligations.

Many inexperienced coaches, pressed for time and unaware of the harm they are doing, go into and through the season winging it from practice to practice. Their argument is simple: They don't have the time to prepare.

You don't need to spend massive amounts of time in preparation for your season and practices. But spending some preparation time will greatly aid your coaching efforts.

Use this chapter to help you prepare for your season and your practices. You will be glad you did—and your players will be, too. Your practices will run more smoothly, with less down time. Your players will learn all they need to learn, and in a logical order. And you will get the most out of your limited time with your players.

Planning Your Season

If you plan from practice to practice without keeping the big picture in mind, you risk overlooking some tactics or skills you should be teaching; you also risk presenting the skills you do teach in less than an ideal order. To make an extreme example, it's no good teaching your players how to pick-and-roll if they can't make basic good passes. It's equally pointless to focus on the outlet pass and fast breaks if your players have no real clues about how to box out and rebound. When you develop a season plan, consider what you should teach throughout the season and when you should teach it.

These three elements will help you construct a plan for your season:

- Purpose
- Tactics and skills
- Rules

Purpose

You should have an overall purpose for every practice, and, when considered in context of the entire season, there should be a logical flow to the purpose of each practice. For example, the purposes in the early-season practices should be to introduce and teach the basic skills. As the season progresses, the purposes should become to refine the basic skills and learn the tactics related to those skills (and to learn more complex skills, if appropriate for the age you're coaching).

Having a purpose gives the practice an informed drive and energy. You and your players are there for a particular reason that day, and your time is spent in trying to accomplish the goals for that practice.

Tactics and Skills

Based on the purpose of the practice, you will focus on teaching a particular skill or tactic. That doesn't mean your players don't practice other tactics or skills during that practice, but that the main emphasis is on learning or refining a particular skill or tactic.

When you lay out, in a season plan, all the skills and tactics you plan to teach, it helps to ensure that you don't overlook something important and that your teaching has a logical flow.

Rules

Many coaches overlook teaching rules to their players. Don't assume your players know the rules. Plan to take some time to teach the basic rules; your players need to know these as much as they need to develop their skills. When you make plans to teach the basic rules, you're much more likely to take the time to do so.

Adjusting Your Season Plan

If you are coaching 6- and 7-year-olds, your season plan will be simpler than if you are coaching 9- and 10-year-olds. As kids gain in size, experience, and physical abilities, they are able to learn more advanced skills and tac-

> **tip**
>
> Teach rules within the context of playing. Set up a block-charge situation in which a player is driving on a defender, briefly explain and demonstrate what movement results in a block and what movement constitutes a charge, and then practice the play. Players learn rules much better in an action context, as opposed to you simply telling them the rules.

tics. In general, keep your plans simple and adjust them as you need to based on your players' abilities. If they've demonstrated they have picked up the basics more quickly than you thought they would, step up your plans a bit. For example, if your 9- and 10-year-olds have demonstrated that they can pretty consistently box out and rebound, take the next step and work on outlet passes and fast breaks.

If, on the other hand, you had planned to work on fast breaks by midseason and your players still haven't mastered the art of boxing out and rebounding, keep your focus on developing those more fundamental skills before moving on to the fast break. And it might be that you never do move on to the fast break that season.

The main point is to adjust your plan to what the players need.

Sample Season Plan

Table 5.1 contains a sample 8-week season plan for a 9- and 10-year-old team that meets once a week. Use it as a guide when you construct your own season plan. Appendix D, "Season Plan," has a blank season plan you can use.

Create your season plan before the season begins. Construct a plan that reflects how many times you will practice throughout the season. Plan your season the way you believe will work best for your players, so long as you cover the basics first and move at a pace that is good for them, adjusting as need be.

Note that you can and should work on multiple skills in a single practice. This model is *not* meant to be the one-and-only way to plan your season; it is one example, intended to give you a start.

Table 5.1   8-week Practice Plan

Week	Focus	Tactics/Skills	Rules
1	Individual offensive skills	**New**: Shooting, passing, dribbling	Double dribble, traveling
2	Individual offensive skills	**New**: Footwork. **Review**: Shooting, passing, dribbling	Pivot foot (traveling)
3	Rebounding, team and individual defense skills	**New**: Establishing position, blocking out, securing the ball. Guarding player with ball, guarding player without ball	Over-the-back foul, fouls on rebounding, reaching in, charging and blocking fouls, allowable defensive contact
4	Team offense	**New**: Screens, pick-and-roll	Legal screens
5	Team offense	**New**: Give-and-go. **Review**: Screens, pick-and-roll	
6	Team defense	**New**: Player-to-player, providing help	
7	Review	Whatever is needed most	
8	Review	Whatever is needed most	

Planning Practices

After you have your season plan in place, you can begin to construct your practice plans. Create your practice plans one at a time—that is, don't create your entire season's worth of practice plans at once because you might find you need to adjust them based on what your players need most to focus on.

This section covers the essential structure of your practices; in "12 Keys to Conducting Effective Practices," we delve into the methods that will help you run successful practices within the structure presented here.

The Best Option: Simultaneous Stations

Basketball coaches have two basic options in structuring their practices. One option is to have all the players together, receiving instruction and then practicing the skills and tactics in one large group. Advantages to this option are that all the players receive the exact same instruction, the coach can easily view the action and provide feedback because only one station is being used, and in practicing team offense and team defense, you necessarily want to play five-on-five.

The downfall is that, for some individual skills, practice time isn't being maximized; players are standing around, waiting for their turn to dribble or shoot. Having only one ball in play and about 10 players is an inefficient way to practice. Players learn and develop their skills less and have more time to goof off.

The better option in teaching individual skills is to run simultaneous stations. After a team warm-up, split the team into two groups and set up two stations. After 15 minutes, instruct the groups to rotate to the other station. In this way, players are active and engaged, they receive more chances to improve their skills, and they're having more fun.

For example, you could set up two separate shooting stations, or you could set up a shooting station at one basket and a dribbling or passing station at the other end of the court.

Simultaneous stations can provide the best learning experiences for players and make practices more active and fun, but they can also present challenges. You need to be aware of those challenges and know how to overcome them. There are two primary challenges: ensuring player safety and maintaining the quality of instruction and feedback provided to players.

Player Safety

Player safety, with simultaneous stations, can be at risk for two reasons: lack of adequate space for setting up the stations and lack of adequate adult supervision. Simply put, don't set up simultaneous stations if you feel that space limitations (perhaps you have only a half court to practice on, for example) or lack of supervision will compromise your players' safety.

As for supervision, the ideal is to have one adult per station. Do you *need* an adult at each station to safely supervise two simultaneous stations? No. Some experienced coaches have safely run simultaneous stations by themselves. In this case, you would set up each station, get players going in each, and move from station to station, observing and providing feedback.

In a better scenario, you will have an assistant coach. (If an assistant hasn't been assigned to you, ask the parents of your players if one or more would like to assist you.

tip

Set up your stations in a way that allows the players at each station to not be infringed upon by play from another station.

tip

Many parents are more than happy to help at practice. Many high school or junior varsity players also enjoy lending a hand at youth practices, whether they have a brother or sister on your team or not. Enlist the help you need to run stations and be clear in how to run the station, which skill execution to look for, and what feedback to give.

Generally, at least one parent will offer to help.) In this way, you could have an adult at each station providing feedback.

Coaching Instruction and Feedback

Of course, the primary purpose of the simultaneous stations is to give players more practice at skill execution. But if Damon continually shoots with an awkward form that is more like a heave as he practices shooting, is he going to improve his shooting skills? Not likely.

Players need feedback on their skill execution. They need to know what's right, what's wrong, and how to fix what's wrong. It's that feedback that helps them learn and improve.

When you have a coach or parent volunteer at each station, you are in the best situation for providing that feedback. Realize, however, that many parents might not know precisely what to look for or what feedback to provide; tell any volunteer exactly what to look for and what type of feedback to give. Give volunteers the easier stations to run, in terms of providing feedback.

Sample Practice Plan

In Appendix E, "Practice Plan," you'll find a blank practice plan you can photocopy and use. See Figure 5.1 for a sample 60-minute practice plan.

Here are a few things to note about the sample plan:

- Instruction time is allotted for each of the stations. You won't always need to allot time for instruction, though. If you have already instructed your players on the skill or tactic, you can start the station with a drill or game.

- Most of the time at a station should be spent in games or drills. You'll learn more about setting up games and drills in "12 Keys to Conducting Effective Practices."

- The Comments section is meant for you to write coaching tips and technique reminders that you want to focus on in that station.

- The Notes section is for things you observe as the players perform at each station. Use this section to jot down observations you want to bring up at the end of practice or techniques you want to work on at the next practice. Use this section to keep a log or journal on your team's progress.

Sample Practice Plan

Date December 15   **Place** McKenzie Gym   **Time** 5:30 p.m.

Equipment balls and pinneys

Purpose   Rebounding and team defense

Activity	Description	Time	Comments
1. Warm-up	Run, stretch, shoot	5-10 min	Focus them on practice purpose
2a.STATION 1: REBOUNDING	*Instruction:* Rebounding	5 min	Positioning, finding your opponent, blocking out, securing the ball
	Game: "Ball Hog"	10 min	1-on-1 and 2-on-2 rebounding drills. Award one point for each rebound and give each player or pair 10 chances on offense to rebound. Then switch defense and offense. Most rebounds wins.
2b. STATION 2: TEAM DEFENSE	*Instruction:* On-the-ball defense	5 min	Positioning, distance from player with ball, use of hands, court awareness
	Drill: "Reaction Drill"	10 min	2-on-2. Player with ball dribbles; defender maintains good positioning and distance. Defender closes up as player picks up dribble and looks to pass. Defense scores 1 point if the offense can't get the ball in the lane within 10 seconds.
2c. STATION 3: TEAM DEFENSE	*Instruction:* Off-the-ball defense	5 min	Denial position and open position
	Game: "Denial"	10 min	2-on-2. Defense gets 1 point if player off the ball can keep her opponent from receiving a pass within 5 seconds, or if the defender intercepts the ball.
3.Wrap-up		5 min	Instructional reminders. Next practice reminder.

Notes

Need more work on getting in finding opponent to block out. Also on maintaining good
positioning in off-the-ball defense and not reaching in on
dribbler.

Conducting Your First Practice

Your first practice is different from all the other practices in a few respects. First, you're probably meeting the majority of your players for the first time, so introductions are in order. Second, you want to create, at the outset, the proper environment, one that balances fun with learning. Your players need to understand that you're there to help them learn and improve their skills. They also need to know what to expect from you and what you expect from them.

You can accomplish this in relatively short order—probably taking 5–10 minutes. From there, you can conduct your practice as normal.

Structure your first practice like this:

1. **Introduction (5–10 minutes)**—Coach and player introductions (kids enjoy a fun icebreaker game here). Goals for the season. Your expectations of players and what they can expect of you. The practice structure. Team rules and safety issues. See the following sidebar, "Setting the Tone," for more detail on this first-practice introduction.

2. **Warm-up (5–10 minutes)**—Light running, stretching, and shooting.

3. **Station 1 (10–15 minutes)**—Shooting instruction and practice. Straight-on shots, side shots, and bank shots.

4. **Station 2 (10–15 minutes)**—Passing instruction and practice. Chest pass and bounce pass.

5. **Station 3 (10–15 minutes)**—Dribbling instruction and practice. Moving forward, weaving through cones, and using the off hand.

6. **Wrap-up (5 minutes)**—Reinforce what most needs to be reinforced, based on activities. Remind players of the next practice or game.

As an alternative, you might consider this structure:

1. Introduction (5 minutes)

2. Warm-up (5–10 minutes)

3. Station 1 (7 minutes)

4. Station 2 (7 minutes)

5. Station 3 (7 minutes)

6. Station 4 (7 minutes)

7. Station 5 (7 minutes)

8. Station 6 (7 minutes)

9. Wrap-up (5 minutes)

In this way, you could work on more skills, albeit for shorter times, and practice would move quickly along.

SETTING THE TONE

To get off on the right foot, you need to communicate certain messages in the first practice and set the tone for a good learning environment. Some things to consider covering in the first practice are

- **Goals for the season**—Briefly tell players your goals for the season, which should be centered on helping them improve their skills, increase their understanding of the game, and have fun.

- **Your expectations**—Let them know that you expect them to show up on time for practice, to pay attention to your instruction and feedback, to obey any rules you set up (mainly concerned with safety), to give full effort, to respect others, to ask questions if they don't understand something, to ask for help when they need it, and to tell you if they are hurt.

- **What players can expect**—Also let players know what to expect from you: that you're there to provide instruction, feedback, and encouragement to help each player improve her skills.

- **Practice structure**—Briefly let players see the big picture of how a typical practice will go.

- **Team rules/safety issues**—Discuss and formulate team rules with players' input. Don't go overboard on rules, but do be clear about safety issues and be strict in enforcing them.

Keep this meeting short, but don't skip over it.

12 Keys to Conducting Effective Practices

At this point you've learned about structuring your season and individual practices. The rest of this chapter is devoted to detailing 12 keys to running effective practices. Here are the keys:

1. Be prepared.
2. Set the stage.
3. Involve parents.
4. Be active.
5. Be active with a purpose.
6. Make it fun.
7. Provide instruction.
8. Give feedback.
9. Be encouraging and supportive.
10. Promote teamwork and camaraderie.

11. Discipline players as necessary.

12. Wrap up the practice.

1. Be Prepared

Sixty minutes—or however long you have for practice—goes by quickly. If you go into practice unprepared, it will go by inefficiently, too.

A little preparation can go a long way. Plan your practice, know what you need to teach, how you want to teach it, which stations you want to run, and which drills or games you want to use to help your players practice their skills. Choose effective drills and games to maximize the learning experience. Be prepared to instruct, give feedback, and provide encouragement.

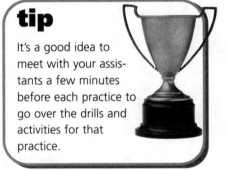

tip

It's a good idea to meet with your assistants a few minutes before each practice to go over the drills and activities for that practice.

That doesn't mean you can't adjust or deviate from your plan. It means you have a plan you can adjust as you need to.

2. Set the Stage

You need to not only have a plan, but also let your players in on that plan. It helps them focus when they know what they're going to practice that day. Let them know the purpose of each practice and the purpose of each drill or game at the practice stations.

How you approach the practice greatly influences your players. If you are cavalier or seemingly uncaring about what happens at practice, your players will follow suit. If you are focused and positive and have a purpose in mind, your players will be more tuned in to the drills and games.

Another way you set the stage is in teaching skills. Don't simply teach the mechanics; let players know why they need to perform the skill, and in what type of situation they will be called upon to perform it in a game. You'll learn more about this in Chapter 6, "Player Development."

3. Involve Parents

Studies show that the more parents are involved in their kids' education, the better their kids do. This shouldn't be too surprising.

Parental involvement has the same effect on youth sport programs, too. But some coaches ward off parents, discouraging their participation. Why? Perhaps because the coaches fear they will lose control of the team when other adults step in or the coaches are concerned that their own lack of knowledge or coaching ability will be revealed. And then there are the few bad-apple parents who are know-it-alls or poor sports or who *do* want to impose their own will at practice. Coaches already have plenty to contend with and can't be blamed for not wanting to deal with this type of parent.

But coaches who steer clear of parental involvement miss out on the advantages that can come with involving them. Here are a few of the roles parents can serve:

> **tip**
>
> Some parents want to help but can't do so at every practice or game. Make it easy for these parents to help by setting up a parent helper rotation. Come up with the ways you need help, find out how many parents are willing to provide that type of help, and set up a rotation for practices and games, so the burden is light and shared.

- **Official or unofficial assistant coaches**—It's extremely helpful to have at least one assistant coach. As noted earlier, it's also helpful to have an adult, whether you call him an assistant coach or a parent aid or whatever, to supervise each station you run at practice. Parents can even help you instruct, if they know the skill and how to teach it.

- **Scorekeepers**—Keeping the scorebook during games is another way parents can help (if you decide you want to keep a scorebook).

- **Drink and snack providers**—Set up a rotation for parents to provide drinks and snacks for games.

- **Special-event planners**—Ask a parent to organize any special event—a pizza party or swimming party—held during the season or for a postseason celebration.

4. Be Active

Simultaneous stations promote continuous, structured activity. Kids can't improve if they have to wait for nine other teammates to practice shooting or rebounding or setting picks. Keep things moving at practice, and don't stay on one point too long. Change the drill or activity every five minutes or so. You can teach the same skill using a different drill or activity, but the child's mind will be more stimulated if it is exposed to two 5-minute drills instead of one 10-minute drill.

5. Be Active with a Purpose

But don't mistake movement and action with purpose. The next worst thing to kids standing around in practice doing nothing is kids bouncing all around the court like balls in a pinball machine with no purpose at all.

When you have prepared for the practice, and when you have set the stage for it and for the games and drills the players are getting ready to participate in, the players' actions are guided by a unified purpose. And when they're guided by that purpose, they are better prepared to learn and hone their skills.

6. Make It Fun

You can have a plan, and you can have a purpose to that plan, but if the practice is dull and boring, filled with repetitive drills that don't seem connected to the actual sport of basketball, you're in trouble. Kids won't pay attention, they won't learn, and they won't care because they're not having fun.

Remember in Chapter 1, "Your Coaching Approach," when you learned about the reasons kids play basketball? The biggest reason they play is that they want to have fun.

Your goal is to teach your players basketball. Their goal is to have fun. When you make your teaching fun, everyone wins.

How do you make practices fun? You've already read about the main way: Keep the kids active. But there's another ingredient, too.

That ingredient is this: Don't practice skills by doing boring, repetitive drills. Practice skills in game-like conditions. This makes it more exciting for your players—and when they need to perform those skills in real games, they'll be more apt to succeed because they've been executing in those same situations in practice. In addition, kids understand the concept of tactics much better when those tactics are introduced and practiced in the context of real-game situations.

Read more about this concept in the following sidebar, "Using Game-like Situations in Practice."

USING GAME-LIKE SITUATIONS IN PRACTICE

Consider ways you could teach the bounce pass. You could have your players pair up, stand 10 to 12 feet apart, and bounce the ball back and forth to each other.

Is there anything innately wrong with this approach? No. It can be useful for practicing the basic technique. But more often than not, in this setup players stand straight-legged, motionless, other than a movement of the arms and a flick of the wrists, producing a weak pass to a stationary teammate.

Don't allow them to do this. Instead, encourage them to *move toward their target* as they pass, to take a step forward, as you would want them to in a game. Have them throw the ball forcefully, but not so hard that it's too hard to handle. Watch their technique. After they have the basics down, put them in two-on-two situations in which the offense must throw only bounce passes to move the ball. If they can complete three passes in a row, or five, or whatever number you decide, the offense "wins." Then switch the offense and defense.

This makes it game-like and fun, and helps the players practice in ways that will translate directly to what they need to do during games.

Be creative. Put kids in game-like situations for all the skills and tactics they practice. When you do, you're doing everyone—including yourself—a favor.

7. Provide Instruction

The next three items on this list—instruction, feedback, and encouragement—are foundational elements in coaching at practice and are closely, and often sequentially, related.

Most coaches realize that to run an effective practice they need to provide quality instruction for their players. But providing good instruction isn't necessarily easy; it's accomplished through a set of learned skills. You'll learn about how to be an effective instructor and teacher of skills in Chapter 6.

8. Give Feedback

After you instruct your players, your coaching duties have just begun. As your players practice the tactics and skills you've taught them, you need to observe their play, assess their technique and understanding, and give them feedback on anything they're doing wrong and on what they should do to improve. How to provide this feedback is also covered in Chapter 6.

9. Be Encouraging and Supportive

All players—from youth leagues through the NBA—need encouragement and support. Basketball is a difficult and challenging game. The skills of the game are not easy to acquire, and even once acquired, they are not easy to consistently execute.

Your players will struggle with picking up the basic skills and with consistently executing them. All players will struggle to improve, regardless of their skill level. You need to nurture their improvement with encouragement and provide a supportive environment for them, and the practice court is the place where this happens. You'll learn specifics of how to provide this encouragement in Chapter 6.

10. Promote Teamwork and Camaraderie

Basketball is a team game. Three-point plays and game-winning shots grab attention, but that game-winning shot might not have been possible without the rebounding ability of your forwards and center, or without the defensive pressure of your guards.

The teams that win are generally more fundamentally sound than other teams. They do the little things right. They maintain good positioning on defense; they box out to rebound; they move without the ball to get open; they see the court and make good passes; they help out on defense as needed.

They know what to do, and more often than not, they are able to do it. They rely on the contributions of many players to win, rather than sitting back and watching one or two teammates do it all.

One of the joys of playing sports is the camaraderie players experience with their teammates. This occurs as players struggle together, as they pull for each other, as they go through wins and losses together, as they exult over individual successes and encourage each other in individual failures, all the while reinforcing the notion that those individual successes and failures are all part of a team effort.

That's how the game and the relationships between players *should* be viewed, and that's the environment you should cultivate. Here are a couple of ideas for cultivating it:

- At the beginning of the season, you or a player's parents could host a pizza and movie night. The players could get together, eat pizza, and watch a basketball movie, such as "Hoosiers."

- At the end of each practice, say something positive about each player. Don't force this; it has to be sincere. If it's too much to say something about every player, single out half of them for compliments at one practice, and address the other half of the team at the end of the next practice. "Way to outlet the ball, Jake," "Nice passing today, Ramon," and "You were picking pockets all day today, Michelle," are examples of the things you might say. When players hear you say something good about everyone, most often for doing small things correctly, it reinforces the team concept.

- Set up a buddy system at practice. Pair up players at each practice and ask that each player pick out something good that his partner did during practice. Switch buddies at each practice so kids get used to encouraging and complimenting different teammates. Again, this exchange shouldn't be forced; emphasize that you want the players to look for good things their teammates do and encourage them to continue to improve.

The main point is to look for ways to emphasize the team aspects of the game and cultivate an environment in which the support and encouragement doesn't just flow from coach to players, but from player to player as well.

11. Discipline Players As Necessary

Part of running an effective practice is to take care of any discipline problems that arise so they don't disrupt the practice.

Even when you conduct a practice that keeps the players active through fun and meaningful drills and games, some kids might misbehave. Here are some suggestions for dealing with different types of misbehavior:

- **Minor misbehavior**—Many times you can ignore minor misbehavior, so long as it doesn't disrupt the practice or distract others from hearing you or from practicing. Kids will sometimes clown around or goof off to draw attention; sometimes if you ignore that behavior, the child will stop it without being told to. If the child *doesn't* stop it and it becomes a distraction to others, you should put a stop to it.

- **Disrespect**—When a player shows disrespect, either to you or to another player, don't let it pass. Use appropriate measures to stop the disrespect.

- **Repeated misbehavior**—If a player is repeatedly misbehaving, even if it's minor misbehavior, you need to address this. Talk to the player, tell him what behavior you need from him, and if the misbehavior continues, punish him appropriately. You might also want to call his parents to let them know of the problem and work together to steer the child toward good behavior.

- **Behavior that puts someone in danger**—You need to put an immediate stop to any behavior that puts someone in danger, and you need to discipline the misbehaving player accordingly.

When you do need to discipline players, do so consistently and impartially. Stick to what you say; if you tell them they will be disciplined for a certain type of behavior and you don't follow through, you're in for trouble.

After you have disciplined a player, don't hold past misbehavior against that player. Also, never discipline a player for making an error, and don't use physical activity—such as running or doing pushups—as a form of punishment. That sends the message that physical activity is bad.

You shouldn't have to discipline your players too much—especially if you keep them engaged in fun activities throughout practice.

12. Wrap Up the Practice

Sixty minutes flies by, and most coaches want to squeeze as much practice as possible out of their time with their players. But it's helpful to take at least a few minutes to wrap up the practice with a brief meeting.

At this meeting, go over what went well, encourage your players (or have them encourage each other, using the buddy system as described earlier), talk about a few things they still need to work on or give constructive feedback based on what you observed in practice, and remind them of the next game or practice. Send the players off with an encouraging word and a smile.

And make sure you're the last to leave the gym, so you know that every player got a ride home.

Then, go home yourself—and plan for your next great practice!

THE ABSOLUTE MINIMUM

This chapter was devoted to helping you construct season and practice plans and to knowing how to run effective practices. Among the key points were

- Make a season plan before your season begins so you can see the big picture of what you want to accomplish. Plan to teach the skills and tactics in a logical order.

- Be willing to adjust your season plan as necessary, based on what your players need.

- Create a practice plan for each practice, one with a specific purpose. Don't forget to teach rules that are related to the skills and tactics you present in that practice.

- At your first practice, let your players know your goals for the season, your expectations of them, what they can expect from you, what the team rules are (as well as the consequences of breaking them), and what the basic practice structure will be.

- Run simultaneous stations in practice so your players are as active as possible. Develop these stations with players' safety in mind.

- Involve parents in running these stations and in other areas where you could use help.

- Focus these stations on fun game-like drills and activities. Players who learn skills in the context of how they should be executed in games are best prepared to execute those skills properly in real games.

- Provide skill instruction, feedback on performance, and encouragement. Cultivate a team atmosphere that promotes camaraderie.

- Discipline players as necessary, following through in appropriate ways that steer the players toward better behavior.

6

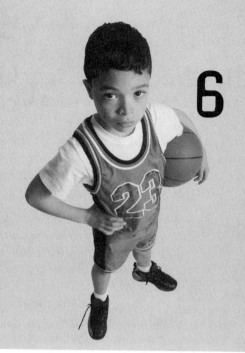

PLAYER DEVELOPMENT

Practice time is all about your players learning and developing the skills and tactics they need to successfully execute in games. And that means you have to be a good teacher, a keen observer, a patient guide, and an encouraging critic.

Sound like a lot? It is, but you can learn how to provide this instruction and guidance. And it's critical that you do because, without it, your players will not fully develop their talents and both you and they will be frustrated.

So get ready to learn how to teach skills and tactics, observe your players, give them the feedback they need, and correct errors. In Chapter 11, "Games and Drills," you'll find games and drills you can use to teach your players the skills and tactics they need to know.

The Process for Teaching Skills and Tactics

"Hey, passing the ball is simple. Even I can do it, and I'm not that good. Why can't they do it?"

"I told them how to set screens. I was concise, clear, and to the point. Why aren't they doing it right?"

"I spent 10 minutes going into detail on how to shoot, but I might as well have been talking to myself, from all the good it did."

Those are among the comments of new coaches, especially if they haven't been in a position to teach before. In the first case, the skill is simple only to the coach, who has likely performed it before. It's not that simple to his players. In the second case, kids need more than an explanation of the skill; they need to see it performed as well. And in the third case, don't mistake the practice court for the lecture hall. Kids don't need a long-winded speech about every minor detail of the skill as it is performed. If you provide one, be prepared for your players to doze off—just as you probably would have at their age.

What *do* your players need? They need you to set the stage for their learning. They need you to show and tell them how to perform the skill or tactic. They need, of course, to practice the skill or tactic. And they need your feedback as they practice.

Set the Stage

The players have just finished warm-ups and Coach Jarvis is ready to practice setting screens. He calls the players over to him, but Jake and Deon continue to throw to each other; they don't hear their coach because they're talking as they warm up.

"All right, guys, we're going to do a three-on-three drill," Coach Jarvis says. Then the coach notices Jake and Deon and calls them over. As they make their way over, Coach Jarvis says, "Let's get six guys out there. Willie, you start with the ball and pass to Zach. All right?"

Had Coach Jarvis been shooting, he would have just missed on three straight attempts. That is, he made three mistakes in setting the stage for this skill instruction:

1. He didn't make sure all his players were listening to him before he began giving instructions.

2. He didn't tell them precisely what they were going to practice.

3. He didn't tell them when or how they would use this skill—whatever it was—in a game.

Why are these things important? Let's look at each issue.

Players' Focus

Coach Jarvis began explaining, in rather cryptic fashion, what the players were going to do before all the players were even within earshot. Even if Coach Jarvis had explained it well, Jake and Deon would have been in the dark about what they were going to be doing.

When you explain a skill or drill to your team, first make sure you have everyone's attention, so practice won't be slowed down as you find yourself explaining things two or three times (see Figure 6.1). Getting your players' attention can sometimes be challenging because two of the main reasons most kids play sports is they want to have fun and they want to hang out with their friends. Put those two together and add in other external and internal distractions, and coaches quickly find that they can't assume their players will always be ready to give them their full attention.

FIGURE 6.1

Get your players' attention before you explain a skill.

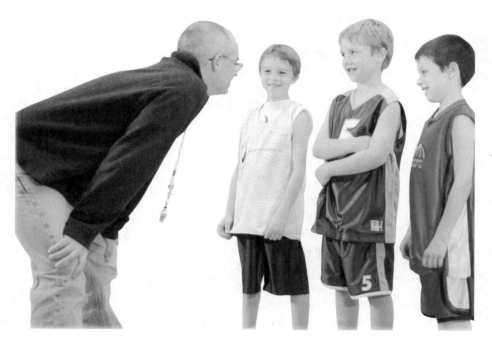

Name That Skill

When you have their attention, identify the skill or tactic you're going to teach. For example, Coach Jarvis should have said something like, "Today we're going to learn how to set screens for our teammates."

Why? For several reasons. First, it gives the players a reference point later. When Coach Jarvis talks about screens, his players will know what he's referring to. For another, it often helps kids get a mental picture of what they're going to be doing. Mainly, though, it helps avoid confusion later. Simply saying, "We're going to do a three-on-three drill" could mean anything; referring to this won't help your players recall anything. "Setting screens for teammates" is explicit and clear and will help them recall the skills involved.

Skill Context

During a league game, Jason receives a pass on the wing after a teammate made a defensive rebound and quick outlet pass. Jason could easily beat all the defenders downcourt and make an uncontested layup, but he dribbles slowly up court, allowing everyone—defenders and teammates alike—to move past him and get into position.

At the next timeout, you ask Jason why he didn't just dribble all the way down and score. "Because you told us not to try to do everything on our own, but to look for our teammates," he replies.

In context, of course, you *do* want your players to look for their teammates. You were making this statement after Willie had been hogging the ball in practice, and missing open teammates. But Jason took your instruction to the extreme and figured he better look for his teammates—even if he could easily score himself.

Many coaches do well in getting their players' attention and in naming a skill or tactic before they begin to teach it, but they don't realize the importance of putting that skill or tactic into context for the players. *You* might understand when the opportunity arises to execute a fast break and exactly how your players should execute it, but your players might not understand these things. And if they don't, chances are they won't successfully execute a fast break when they get the chance.

To help them understand, you could ask a few questions such as, "After you get a rebound, what should you look to do next?" "What players should you look to outlet the ball to?" "Where should the other players go?" "What lanes should they fill on a fast break?"

If you receive a correct answer to one of your questions, make sure everyone heard it and understands it before moving on. If you're not sure whether everyone heard or understands, or if no one gave a correct answer, give a brief, clear answer yourself—something like, "After you get a rebound, you should look to make an outlet pass to a teammate—preferably one of the guards. This can help us get a fast break going and get a good scoring opportunity."

tip

To get your players' attention, call them together and make eye contact with each one. If some aren't looking at you, call their names so you make eye contact. Wait until the players are quiet and attentive. If this doesn't happen within a few moments, ask them to stop talking, look at you, and give you their full attention. Don't go on until they do so.

You might even make this rule at the beginning of the season: Whenever you hear two short blasts on my whistle, everyone races to mid-court, sits down, and gives their full attention to me.

Don't take long with your explanations, but do be clear about how to execute the skill and why it is important to the team. Let your players know how the team benefits when the skill or tactic is correctly executed.

Show and Tell

Naming the skill and putting it in context should take just a few moments. The next step, show and tell, will take a little longer.

Some inexperienced coaches make the mistake of *telling* their players how to perform a skill but not *showing* them how. A verbal explanation isn't enough. Neither is just a visual demonstration. If you briefly explain the skill as you demonstrate it, it should sink in (see Figure 6.2).

For example, in teaching how to make a bounce pass, you should *tell* your players how to hold the ball in both hands, take a step toward their target, crisply bounce the ball so that it lands about two-thirds of the way toward their target, and bounce it so that it comes to the teammate's midsection, while *you are showing* them how to do everything you said. The visual demonstration is vital to their comprehension.

note

One of the joys of coaching is when you see your players respond correctly in a situation without telling them what to do. When you put tactics and skills in context of how they're used in a game, your players will learn not just the tactic or skill, but the game itself.

FIGURE 6.2

Explain the skill as you demonstrate it.

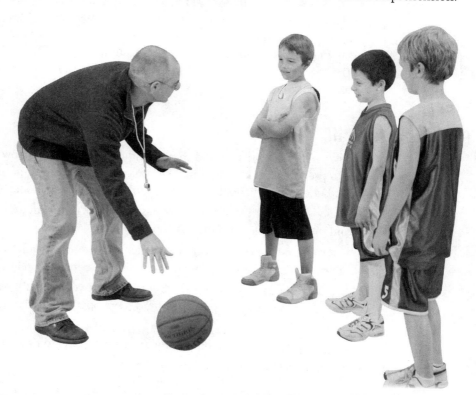

Here are a few pointers on what to say about a skill and how to demonstrate it.

What to say:

- Briefly and clearly explain the technique. You should be able to explain the technique for most skills in no more than a minute or two.
- Use language your players understand.
- To see if your players understand what to do, ask them how they are going to perform the skill after you're finished explaining and demonstrating it.

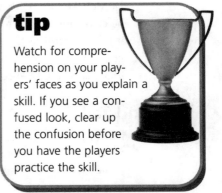

tip

Watch for comprehension on your players' faces as you explain a skill. If you see a confused look, clear up the confusion before you have the players practice the skill.

What to show:

- Perform the skill as you talk your way through it.
- Show the skill a few times.
- If necessary, use an assistant coach, a parent, or a player to help you demonstrate a skill. You might need to use someone else either to show correct form or to show how two players execute a tactic.
- Break a skill into parts, showing each part first and then showing the complete skill without a break. For example, on a rebound, show good defensive positioning and how to locate the player you're defending to make sure you are in good position to block out. Then show good technique in blocking out. Then show how to go after, and secure, the rebound. Finally, show the complete skill all at once.

Practice the Skill

After you've introduced a skill and shown and told your players how to perform it, have them practice the skill in game-like situations. Use drills or games that simulate the experiences they will have in real games and observe their techniques.

Here are suggestions for constructing games and drills that simulate real-game situations and maximize player participation:

- Use the simultaneous-station idea when appropriate. Look to create as many opportunities as possible for each player to practice the skill.
- Use controlled drills and scrimmages in which you set up plays and have each team execute the plays, keeping score based on their successful executions.
- Focus the action on the skill you want your players to practice, with as little other action surrounding that skill execution as possible. Take care, though, to keep the action realistic, not cutting off too much.

■ As noted in Chapter 5, "Practice Plans," you should make the games and drills fun. Score them in some way, make them competitive, or add a twist to them while maintaining their realism.

■ Construct each game around a singular, clear purpose. Directly tie in to the purpose the successful execution of the skill or tactic.

■ Consider ways to make the games a little easier for less talented players and a little harder for more skilled players.

■ Make the games simple to explain and understand. You don't want to spend five minutes explaining the game and spend additional time re-explaining it as the players play.

Be sure to see the sample games and drills in Chapter 11.

Provide Feedback

As players take part in a drill or game, practicing the skill or tactic you've just taught them, observe their execution and be ready to provide feedback to help them correct errors and improve their play. In this section, you learn about feedback content, timing, whether you should alter your feedback for athletes of varying abilities, and what to do for the kids who just don't seem to get it.

Feedback Content

Focus most of your feedback on the players' attempts to execute the skill you just taught. Don't overload them with feedback as they practice, but do give your shooters coaching cues, such as, "Square your shoulders!" or "Use your legs!" Similar cues to your defenders guarding players without the ball might be, "Denial position!" "Watch the passing lane!" These comments are short enough not to distract them and should serve as reminders of the technique you just taught.

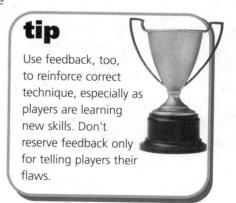

tip

Use feedback, too, to reinforce correct technique, especially as players are learning new skills. Don't reserve feedback only for telling players their flaws.

However, that doesn't mean you can't provide some feedback concerning related skills. Maybe you're practicing fast breaks and you notice your players have a tendency to charge into the defender at the other end. You can provide coaching cues such as, "Pull up and pass it!" or "Under control!"

Feedback Timing

In most cases, the best time to give feedback is as soon as you see something you should comment on, either affirming correct technique or helping a player improve incorrect technique. Many times, as mentioned, you can use coaching cues to remind players of correct technique; you can give these cues as they are participating in the drill or game without stopping the flow.

You can also provide feedback at the end of the drill, game, or practice, especially if what you have to say applies to multiple players.

If you have feedback that really applies only to one player, in addition to giving feedback on the spot, you can also draw that player aside after the drill or at the end of practice and give him your feedback.

If several of your players are having difficulty performing the skill you just taught and they appear not to know how to go about it, you need to stop the action and reteach the skill. There was a disconnection between your teaching and their learning, and you need to teach the skill in a way that is clear to them—or ask yourself if the skill is too advanced for their ability level. If that's the case, perhaps you need to keep your players focused on refining the fundamental skills.

Altering Your Feedback

Theo, Albert, and Chris are guards on your team.

Theo is a natural on the court. He is quick and fluid, he is a very good ballhandler, he "sees" the court well, and he has a knack for making the right play at the right time. Theo is a tough kid, a quiet but focused leader. He doesn't like to make mistakes, but when he does, he shakes them off.

Albert has some talent, but he is a year younger than Theo, and his talent is raw. He is inconsistent with his mechanics and appears lackadaisical at times, half-heartedly playing defense while waiting for his next opportunity on offense.

Chris has limited talent, but he loves the game, tries hard, and gets down on himself when he makes mistakes or doesn't make plays he thinks he should have. Chris is the least-skilled of the three, though he's more consistent than Albert.

Do you provide the same type of feedback to your three guards? Let's say that in similar situations, with each guard controlling the ball near the top of the key, these things happen:

- Theo sees Tyler flash across the middle, hits him with a perfect pass, and Tyler scores.
- Albert sees Tyler flash across the middle, ignores him, puts up a shot while he is well-defended, and misses badly.
- Chris sees Tyler flash across the middle, passes to him, and has the pass intercepted.

With Theo, you tell him, "Way to go!" But what about Albert and Chris? They had a similar outcome in that they failed to make the desirable play (the pass to Tyler), but you feel Albert selfishly chose not to pass and made a bad decision in taking a long, contested shot, while Chris made the right decision but just wasn't able to execute the pass.

You should applaud Chris for his efforts and encourage him, and you should exhort Albert to look for the open player, while not shaming him in front of his team-mates.

The point is that you will be giving feedback on effort, mental approach, and team play, as well as physical technique. You will be giving feedback to players with a lot of talent, players who have minimal talent, and players who vary in their desires for the game and their emotional makeup.

Shape your feedback to best help the player improve his abilities to play the game. Don't panic; this doesn't mean you have to have a different approach for every player. It just means you need to consider what type of feedback will best help the player improve.

Theo and Chris likely won't need any encouragement from you to give it their all. They *will* likely need feedback on technique, but you shouldn't expect Chris to per-form at the same level as Theo, so your feedback will be tempered by that and by your understanding that he's hard on himself. You want to focus your feedback on the technical aspects of courting and give all your players—especially those who, like Chris, are hard on themselves—plenty of encouragement.

As you get to know your players, this tailoring of feedback becomes relatively sim-ple. For now, be aware that, just as your players are individuals, you should shape your feedback according to their individual needs, all with the same end goal in mind—to help them improve their skills.

If at First a Player Doesn't Succeed...

...*don't* ask her to just "try, try again," even though that's how the saying goes. Instead, ask yourself why the player is failing.

Why ask this question? Because a player can make a mistake for many reasons, and the reason should affect how you respond. Here are some of the reasons:

- The player doesn't know the correct technique.
- She knows the correct technique but doesn't understand the rules or the spe-cific strategy called for.
- She doesn't appear to be giving her full effort.
- She is too anxious about her performance.

Let's consider how you should respond in each situation.

If a player is making mistakes because she doesn't know the correct technique, she doesn't need your encouragement; she needs your instruction on the mechanics of the skill.

If a player knows the correct technique but makes a mistake because she's not sure what to do, you need to clarify the rules or explain the strategy called for in that situation.

If a player makes a mistake or doesn't make a play because of a lack of desire or effort, you need to talk privately with the player and find out why she is giving less than full effort. You should work with the player to eradicate the problem and encourage her to give full effort at all times, both for herself and for her teammates.

If a player is making mistakes because she is overanxious about her performance, you should talk with this player privately and help her put her performance in perspective. If the anxiety continues, consider moving her to a different position, or using her differently in your game plan, with the intent of taking pressure off of her. Help her focus on the technical, physical aspects of the game.

What if a player knows the correct technique, knows the rules and strategies involved, is giving full effort, and isn't overly anxious about her performance, but she still makes lots of mistakes?

This youngster needs two things: practice and encouragement. Provide all the opportunities you can for her in practice, and suggest to her parents that they might work with her at home on her skills.

Six Keys to Mistake Correction

You've heard the saying, "Practice makes perfect." Well, if practice made perfect, NBA players would never commit a turnover. Although practice certainly helps players improve, you will have plenty of technical flaws and other types of mistakes to correct. Here are six keys to correcting mistakes:

1. Be encouraging.
2. Be honest.
3. Be specific.
4. Reinforce correct technique.
5. Explain why the mistake happened.
6. Watch for comprehension.

Let's consider each key.

Be Encouraging

Players are usually discouraged when they make a poor play. They need to be corrected, but they also need to be encouraged.

Look for something you can praise, even as you prepare to correct the player. Commend him for his effort. Acknowledge something he did correctly: "Way to spot your open teammate, Chris." After you have corrected his technique, end with a smile and a word of encouragement.

Be Honest

Be encouraging, yes, but don't be dishonest. Don't say, "Nice form, Nick!" if Nick's form leaves much to be desired. False praise isn't going to help Nick; honesty and correction are.

And don't falsely praise some inconsequential thing, just to give some praise. Kids see through that, and if they know you're not leveling with them, they will be insulted and might question more legitimate comments you make. For example, suppose Robby zings an outlet pass over a team-mate's head and you, in trying to say something positive, blurt out, "Way to zing the ball out there, Robby!" Robby will either think you're making fun of him or know you're reaching for a compliment because he threw the pass poorly. Nothing about the pass could be realistically complimented. You *could*, however, compliment Robby for blocking out his opponent and snaring the rebound, and then tell him how to correct his passing.

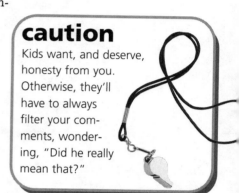

caution

Kids want, and deserve, honesty from you. Otherwise, they'll have to always filter your comments, wondering, "Did he really mean that?"

Be Specific

When you correct faulty technique, be specific. During shooting practice, don't say, "Come on, Andi! We need you to shoot better than that!" That doesn't help Andi know what she's doing incorrectly. Rather, say, "Andi, you're holding the ball on the palm of your hands. Try releasing it off your fingertips. You can do it."

Focus your correction on the technical aspects the player needs to change, being clear and specific in your comments. Keep your feedback short and precise, and remember to demonstrate the correct action to reinforce your verbal message (see Figure 6.3).

Reinforce Correct Technique

Ben receives a pass and is open for what should be a short bank shot about six feet from the basket. He stands flat-footed and shoots straight at the basket, not using the backboard. He misses the shot.

Some inexperienced coaches would show Ben just what he did wrong: He stood flat-footed, and he shot at the rim, not at the backboard. And, assuming they had taught Ben how to shoot before, they would be wasting their time.

Why? Because Ben already knows he used incorrect technique. You don't need to demonstrate what he did wrong; he already attempted to shoot that way. He needs to see what he *should* do.

FIGURE 6.3
Be clear and
specific in cor-
recting errors.

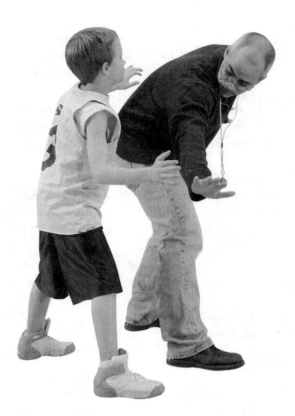

Many times, even if you say, "Don't do it this way," or "Here's what you did wrong," as you show the incorrect technique, the player does not hear the message or the incorrect technique is reinforced in his mind's eye because he's seeing it all over again.

Simply show him how to correctly perform the technique, tell him what to do, and let him try it again.

Explain Why the Mistake Happened

Sometimes kids don't understand what they're doing wrong. You can briefly explain it, without demonstrating the incorrect technique. This explanation can help them understand what they're doing wrong and, as you tell and show them how to execute the skill correctly, they are more likely to get it if they understand what to change.

For example, if Tara often gets the ball stolen from her while she dribbles, tell her that she's not protecting the ball from her opponent and she's bouncing the ball too high. Then tell and show her how to use her body to protect the ball while she's dribbling, and how to dribble lower.

Most often, however, your players will not need much of an explanation for why they committed the mistake. Focus most of your time on explaining and demonstrating correct technique.

Watch for Comprehension

Earlier you read about the need to watch for comprehension on your players' faces as you teach them a new skill. You need to watch for this same comprehension as you correct their technique, too.

Look for understanding in your players' eyes and if there's any doubt, ask them, "Do you understand what I mean?" If they don't, couch your verbal message differently, making sure your demonstration of the technique is clear as well.

The effectiveness of your correction is not based on how clear your message is to you; it's based on how well it's received by your players.

THE ABSOLUTE MINIMUM

This chapter focused on your approach to teaching skills and tactics and correcting mistakes. Key points to remember include

- Remember the method to teaching skills: Set the stage for your players' learning, use a show-and-tell approach to teaching, practice the skill, and provide feedback.

- In setting the stage, make sure your players are listening, name the skill, and put it in context for your players so they can see how they will use it in a game and how correct execution of the skill will benefit the team.

- In the show-and-tell phase, briefly and clearly explain and demonstrate the skill. Watch for player comprehension as you do this, and be ready to clear up any confusion.

- Break down a skill in parts, showing the whole skill, then each individual part alone, and then perform the entire skill again.

- Provide clear feedback to help players improve their skills.

- Consider reasons why players are making mistakes and tailor your feedback accordingly. Sometimes they might not know how to perform the skill and need skill instruction; at other times they might understand how to perform the skill but need help improving their mechanics. They also might not understand the rules or strategies that relate to the situation.

- When correcting mistakes, keep these six keys in mind: Be encouraging, be honest, be specific, reinforce correct technique, explain why the mistake happened, and watch for comprehension.

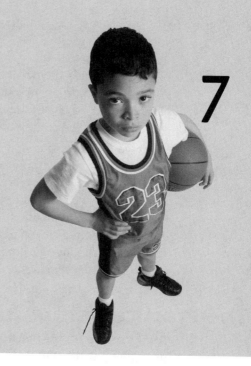

7

Game Time!

The gym begins to fill with parents, grandparents, and siblings of players. The players arrive singly and in pairs, looking crisp and sharp in their uniforms. As they warm up, you can see the excitement in their faces.

A few butterflies stir to life in your stomach. For every butterfly fluttering in your stomach, you figure there must be a dozen in your players' bellies. Anticipation, hope, anxiety, and joy intermingle in the air. In a few minutes, the referee will stride to the center circle, the starters from both teams will align themselves along the circle, with two inside the circle to contest the jump ball, the referee will make the toss, and the game will begin.

There's nothing like game time, nothing like that opening jump ball, releasing the tension that has been building since the first players arrived for warm-ups.

Playing games is really what it's all about. Kids come to practice to learn and hone skills with one purpose in mind: To play as well as possible during games. It takes planning and expertise to make practices fun, but playing league games is *inherently* fun and is the main reason that most kids sign up to play.

So far, you've learned to apply the keys to coaching to your practices. In this chapter you learn to apply those keys before, during, and after games. What should you communicate to your players at the practice before a game? When the game rolls around, do you change your approach to coaching in any way? How should you rotate players in and out? How much teaching and mistake correction should you do during a game? How much strategy should you employ during a game? What should you tell players before and after a game? For the answers to these and many similar questions, read on.

The Practice Before the Game

For the most part, the practice immediately preceding a game will not differ from any other practice. But there are a few things you need to discuss with your players, including the game particulars and the team's tactical focus for the game.

Game Particulars

At the end of the practice, remind the players of the game time, the gym location, and what time you want them to arrive at the gym to warm up. Tell them to arrive 20 minutes before the game so they have enough time to warm up. Remind them to wear their team uniforms and bring their water bottles.

Give your players some guidance on what to eat, what not to eat, and how soon before a game they should eat. See the following sidebar, "Fueling Up," for guidelines on what players should eat and drink before, during, and after games.

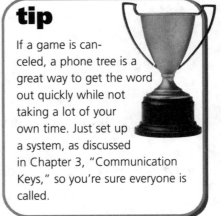

tip

If a game is canceled, a phone tree is a great way to get the word out quickly while not taking a lot of your own time. Just set up a system, as discussed in Chapter 3, "Communication Keys," so you're sure everyone is called.

FUELING UP

It's 20 minutes before game time. Do you know what's in your players' stomachs? Whatever it is, they will use it as the fuel in their tanks for the game.

Hopefully, their fuel doesn't consist of a big steak dinner or a couple of fast-food burgers lathered in "special" (read *fat-laden*) sauce, with a large order of fries, washed down with a soft drink.

Why? Because foods high in fat take longer to digest. Your players should have easily digested food in their stomachs, so their energy goes toward playing rather than digesting. The carbonation in soft drinks can cause indigestion, and the sugar content results in a rise in blood insulin levels, which can make players tired. Tell your players not to have soft drinks within a few hours of a game.

That doesn't mean they should show up empty-stomached. That's like taking off on a drive with your gas tank all but dry.

Players should have something light and digestible an hour or two before the game—a bagel or toast and a little fruit would be good, though a lot of fruit can cause gastrointestinal stress. Some cereal to tide them over until after the game works, too.

If they have time, they can eat a light meal two to three hours before the game. This meal should be high in carbohydrates and low in fat.

As for fluids, players should drink water before, during, and after a game. Sports drinks are good, too, and provide the added benefit of replacing minerals and electrolytes lost through exercise and sweat. Players should drink 2 or 3 cups of water or sports drink (24–30 ounces) within two hours of a game and drink about 8 ounces of fluid every 20 minutes during a game.

After a game, they should continue to rehydrate and eat a meal high in carbohydrates.

Game Focus

Your team's tactical focus might consist solely of executing the fundamentals well—and if your team does that, it has an excellent chance of winning. Especially at younger levels of play (say, six–nine years old), there isn't much need for intricate tactics; you want your players to simply focus on executing the individual skills well.

At the younger levels, your strategy should be easily remembered, with much or all of it becoming part of your season-long mantra: "Move the ball. Look for the open player. Take good shots. Block out and rebound. Play good defense."

If you are coaching older or more experienced players, however, you can and should consider your tactical approach to the game. This approach hinges on your players' strengths and abilities and on the opponent you're facing.

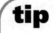

tip

Don't just dictate team strategy for older players; ask their input. This helps them to consider their strengths and the strategies that would help them win. It also results in them perhaps more fully buying into the strategies because they had a part in designing them.

What are some of the tactical approaches you might consider?

- ■ **Use a full-court press**—This is good to do if you have quick, able defenders (although realize that some younger leagues don't allow full-court presses).

- ■ **Dribble penetration**—This works if you have a good, quick ballhandler who can drive to the basket and either get a good shot or draw the defense to him and pass off to an open teammate nearby.

- ■ **Pass it back out**—If you have good perimeter shooters, one tactic to get them open shots is to pass the ball down low or into the middle, in or near the lane. Then, as the defense sags in to help, the pass goes back out to a player left open for a shot.

- ■ **Zone defense**—In a zone, each defender covers a certain portion of the court. This can be a good choice if the team you're playing is much quicker than you are, if they are poor outside shooters, or their primary strategy is to penetrate by the dribble.

- ■ **Player-to-player defense**—In this defense, each defender is assigned to guard a single opponent. This is generally easier for kids to remember, and is recommended unless the other team is significantly quicker than your team.

- ■ **Running game**—A *running game*, meaning a team looks to fast break as often as possible, is most effective with at least one player who can make accurate outlet passes and other players who are quick and sure ballhandlers. It's especially good to use if your team has superior speed and quickness.

- ■ **Slow tempo game**—If you're playing an opponent who has a quickness and ability advantage over your team, you can counter that advantage by slowing the pace of the game, being deliberate in how you move the ball up the court and look for shots. In reality, this type of game is rarely seen at the youth level, but it's a strategy that can be employed at the older levels, as players develop patience and court sense.

Before the Game

Arrive about 30 minutes before game time, if possible. Use the 10 minutes or so that you have before your players arrive to check the court for any hazards. In addition to checking the court, you have three other duties to tend to before the game begins: making sure your team warms up properly, figuring out your starting lineup, and giving your players a few pearls of wisdom before they take to the court.

Team Warm-up

This is simple enough, and players should know the routine from practice. They need to jog a few minutes, stretch, and do a few light drills that focus on some of the skills they will be performing: shooting, passing, and dribbling. You can combine some of the jogging and shooting by having them form two layup lines. Make sure they also practice the other types of shots they will take in the game.

Starting Lineups

Starting lineups can be tricky to concoct if players show up just a few minutes before game time, or not at all. If you've figured out your starting lineup at home, be ready to change it at the last minute.

If you plan to play everyone an equal amount of time, as is often the case at younger levels of competition, there's not a tremendous amount of difference in figuring out your lineup; you just have to figure out how to get everyone in. This issue is addressed later in this chapter. At older levels, as you play your better players more, some strategy does come into play in making out your starting lineup.

In "Player Substitutions" later in this chapter, you'll consider options in rotating players in and out of the lineup, in rotating players at various positions, and in playing time issues.

note

Many coaches have various starting lineups in mind: their quick team, their big team, their best offensive team, and their best defensive team. Depending on the game situation, these units will play together. A player might not be on the court to start the game, but if he knows he's on the starting defensive team and is essentially a starter in crucial defensive situations, this gives him an identity and is a great morale builder.

Last-Minute Words

As noted in Chapter 3, you don't need to fire up your troops with a dramatic pep talk. But you do need to help them prepare to compete, and a few well-chosen words before the game can do just that.

Remind them to focus on the basics and to execute the fundamental skills and tactics they have been practicing. Go over any particular strategies or game plans you discussed in the previous practice. You might also note how you will substitute players in, although you don't necessarily need to divulge this. Sometimes, however, it's easy enough to let players know the general approach to when and how they will be subbed in, and this can help them get mentally prepared.

Above all, tell them to play hard and have fun.

Your talk might go something like this: "All right, guys, let's look for the open player. Move the ball around, look for good shots, and remember to block out and rebound after that ball goes up. Be aggressive! Play tough defense. Let's play hard, play smart, and have fun. Are you ready?"

This will help focus your players on the fundamentals, remind them of the game plan, and keep the big picture in mind.

During the Game

You know your role as coach at practice and how to plan for practices and run them effectively.

But what, if anything, changes for you during games? Does your coaching role change? Is there a subtle shift in your approach? Do you do the same amount and type of coaching? How do you respond to players' mistakes, and how do you plan to rotate your players in and out?

This section takes a look at your role as coach during the game, providing strategies and tips to help you effectively guide your players throughout the contest.

Your Approach to the Game

During every practice, your focus is on helping your players acquire and develop the physical skills, tactical abilities, and mental approach and understanding to do what? To compete, with the goal of winning clearly in mind. Winning is the common goal of every team. Your job is to prepare your players in a way that puts them in a position to compete and to win.

Your job is also, as stated in Chapter 1, "Your Coaching Approach," to not overemphasize winning. Or, more directly put, you need to emphasize player development over winning. Of course, when you emphasize this development, you increase your chances of winning, so you're not working against yourself or your players here.

This all sounds so much easier than it really is. The pressure to win is enormous, and the inclination among players and coaches alike is to define themselves according to their win-loss record or personal achievements.

If you approach the game in a way that reinforces that winning-is-everything mentality in players' minds, you are doing them a disservice. If your coaching decisions reflect your concern first for your players and their development, and then your desire to win, you have the right approach. But you have to consciously go into each game with this mindset because the common mindset runs contrary to this.

Other considerations in your approach include how much coaching you do, what type of coaching you provide, how you employ strategies in your game plan, and how you address or correct mistakes during games. Let's examine these issues one at a time.

How Much Coaching?

How much coaching you do during a game depends on what your players need. You don't want to over-coach, and you don't want to under-coach.

Some of the signs of over-coaching include

- You have a thick playbook denoting all the variables of the offenses and defenses you want to employ, and most NBA players would have difficulty understanding this playbook.

- You prepare and rehearse a five-minute pep talk aimed solely at "firing up" the troops.

- You never stop talking throughout the game. You constantly give instructions about how to shoot, pass, dribble, rebound, and defend.

- When a player makes a mistake, you substitute for her and give her detailed skill instruction on the sideline.

- You spend hours analyzing your team's statistics after games.

- You get all over the 16-year-old referee because you think he missed a borderline call.

- You send a scout to watch your next opponent's practice.

- You contest a foul called on one of your players, even though you see that your player clearly committed the foul, in hopes of "softening up" the referee for other calls later in the game.

Almost as bad as over-coaching is under-coaching. Some of the signs of under-coaching include

- You don't tell your players what to focus on before the game begins; you simply show up, name the starters, wish your players "Good luck," and settle in to watch the game.

- You don't provide any brief coaching tips or cues to your players.

- When a player asks you for some specific guidance, you just clap your hands and say, "Do your best."

- You give no encouragement to your players.

- One of your players is losing his cool and is on the borderline of being thrown out of the game, and you don't intervene.

- One of your players is upset about a mistake he has made, and he sits in tears on the bench as you sit, passive and mute, a few feet away.

- One of your players is overmatched against an opponent and is being scored upon nearly every time her opposing player touches the ball. You leave your player in, and don't switch defensive assignments, because that's the assignment you made for her before the game.

Some extreme examples are in both of those lists, but they aren't so extreme, unfortunately, as to be rare. What you should aim for is something that falls between over- and under-coaching. What's the right amount of coaching in youth basketball? Here are seven keys to coaching effectively during games:

- **Help your players get mentally prepared**—Remind them of their focus for the game and of any game plan you devised in the previous practice. Keep them zoned in on properly executing the fundamentals. They will have nervous energy; you need to help them direct and expend that energy in ways that will help them compete well.

- **Provide tactical direction**—Guide your players in the appropriate tactics as situations arise. Don't expect them to automatically know what to do in each situation. Let them know you want to put greater pressure on the guards on defense, or run the fast break, or look to get the ball down low because the opponents' interior defense is weak. And remember, don't ask them to do something in a game that they haven't practiced!

- **Be involved, and be encouraging**—Part of being involved happens as you provide that tactical direction. Stay in the game mentally and emotionally. Encourage your players, and foster that same type of support among the players themselves.

- **Give technique tips and reminders**—Don't go into full-blown, detailed instruction on skills; save that for the next practice if you see that players are not executing correctly. Giving too much instruction during a game takes a player's focus off the game itself. But *do* give technique tips and reminders, cues that will help them remember what you taught them in practice: "Follow through on your shots!" "Box out!" "Protect the ball!" "Don't reach in!" These technique tips should be enough to remind them of the more complete instruction you gave at previous practices.

> **tip**
>
> To provide helpful tips that don't distract your players, keep them short, clear, specific, and related directly to what you have previously taught.

- **Let the players play**—Guide your players, yes, but don't be like a puppeteer with invisible strings attached to them, prompting their every move. It's your duty to teach them the skills and tactics and to let them experience the game as they compete against other teams. You coach and direct during games, but not with such a heavy hand that your players can't, or don't want to, think for themselves. Part of the joy for the players is learning how to perform and make decisions in games. Beyond ensuring that all your players get in the game, don't make numerous personnel moves, and don't constantly shout out instructions. Keep in the game, give players technique tips and encouragement, and let them play.

- **Tend to your players' needs**—Letting your players play doesn't mean you don't tend to their needs. Remind them before the game of your tactical approach or game plan. Give them coaching tips, support, and encouragement. If a player is disconsolate, tend to him; if a player twists an ankle, tend to her. Provide general direction throughout the game. And supply one more thing, which is the final item in this list.

- **Help your players keep the proper perspective**—Many coaches provide essentially everything their players need, except for this last item: Keeping the game in perspective. These coaches build up each game as if it's an NBA Finals encounter and celebrate wins excessively while moping or grousing about the referees in defeat. Their players, of course, tend to take their cues from these coaches. The players make more of victories than they should, and they are poor sports or depressed in defeat, sulking or obsessing over a play they could have made that might have turned the game around.

    Don't do this to your players! Don't make more of a victory than it is because then kids get too wrapped up in the game's outcome, which they can't control. Keep them focused on their performances, which they *can* control. Even in victory, there are things to improve, and even in defeat, there are successes to be found. Help your players enjoy the game, to play it hard and as well as they can, and to learn from both wins and losses, while keeping both in proper perspective. It is, after all, a game. And it should be left on the court, win or lose. Young hearts and minds shouldn't labor long over a loss, and young heads shouldn't become so large after a win that players have difficulty pulling off their shirts when they get home.

Positive Coaching

Imagine Coach Swanson, in irritation or anger, shouting these comments during a game, for everyone (his players, opposing players, and fans) to hear:

> "Come on, Nathan! How many times have I told you not to go for those head fakes?"

> "Lucas! What kind of shot is that? You are *not* shooting how I taught you to shoot!"

> "Ann, you have to put some zip on that ball! They stole it because you made a weak pass!"

Chances are pretty good that Nathan, Lucas, and Ann will play the rest of the game with one eye on their coach, hoping not to make another play that draws Coach Swanson's ire or derogatory comments.

There's something about public humiliation that makes kids tentative.

Yet way too many coaches publicly humiliate their players, either consciously or unconsciously. These are the same coaches who attach too much importance to winning, who conveniently forget to put in their least-skilled players (or put them in for a token minute or two), and who grouse all game long at the referees.

It would have been far more appropriate if Coach Swanson had, at an opportune moment, privately and calmly given Nathan, Lucas, and Ann the brief technique tip he or she needed, along with an encouraging pat on the back, before sending him or her back out on the court.

Look to build up your players, not tear them down. Teach in a positive manner, and keep control of your own emotions. Keep your comments focused on the techniques players need to improve, delivering them in a way that lets players know you are on their side. Remind them of times in the past when they performed the skill well. Help them to see themselves successfully performing it, and show by your words and body language that you believe they can do it again.

caution

Remember, if your body language belies your words—if you say, "You can do it," but your shoulders are sagging and you look irritated or disbelieving—the player will not believe your positive words.

Appropriate Strategy

Again, at the younger levels, your main strategy is to have your players execute the fundamentals. As the players gain in age, size, experience, and ability, you can begin to employ various strategies to help your team win. And, as noted earlier, when you involve your players in some of these strategy decisions and they have input into the game plan, they enjoy the game more, develop their ability to understand the mental and tactical aspects of the game, and feel more of a buy-in to the plan. It therefore helps them develop as players.

Put your players in situations where they are most likely to succeed and where they are most talented. If your players aren't as quick as the other team, don't try to press or play an overly tight defense. If your players aren't good outside shooters, don't emphasize three-pointers or longer shots. Keep your strategy in line with your players' skill levels and the game situation.

Minimal Mistake Correction

Your players are going to make mistakes. So much of coaching is helping players correct mistakes. How should you approach this duty during games?

First, note the types of mistakes that are made by more than one player. You should address the necessary skill execution for the entire team in your next practice.

Second, note mistakes made by individual players. Perhaps Bobby dribbles too high and leaves the ball exposed to his defender. Maybe Matt doesn't move his feet well enough to get in good rebounding position, or moves his pivot foot and is often called for traveling. Give Bobby and Matt brief instruction during the game, reminding them of the proper techniques they have been taught.

Games are for playing, not for detailed instruction. Your players' focus should be on the game. Save the more detailed instruction and technique practice for your next practice.

Player Substitutions

There are two issues to consider as you plan your player substitutions: playing time and in-game substitutions. Let's take a look at each issue.

Playing Time

Is equal playing time appropriate? Is it fair? Should your less talented players play as much as your more talented players?

The first question to answer is actually this one: Does your league require equal playing time? Some leagues do, and some don't. Often, as the kids get older, this requirement—if in place at all—is dropped.

If it is in place, you need to have a plan that results in your players getting the same number of minutes.

If it's not in place, you need to decide whether you think an equal playing time policy is fitting. There are two camps of thought here. They go something like this:

- **For equal playing time**—"The outcome of the game isn't as important as it is for the players to develop their skills and have fun. How are the lesser-skilled players going to develop their skills if they don't play? And what's the fun of sitting on the bench?"

- **Against equal playing time**—"Why punish the better players by sitting them down, and why risk losing by playing your lesser-skilled players as much as your more talented athletes? That's not teaching the kids realistic lessons about competition, anyway, because in all other aspects of life, the emphasis is on winning and the attitude is dog-eat-dog."

Equal playing time makes sense, whether it's league policy or not, for players eight years old and younger. After that, playing time should shift more and more to the better players, though lesser-skilled players should still get decent chunks of playing time at ages 9 and 10. By 11 and 12, most of the playing time normally goes to the better athletes.

The main point here is to think out your plan before you get to the court. Know not only who you plan to start, but when and how you plan to substitute.

In-Game Substitutions

One of your game responsibilities is to make substitutions. At the earlier ages, make your substitutions to ensure all players get about equal playing time. The easiest situation here is if you have 10 players; each player would play half the game. You could have one group of players play the first and third quarters and another group play the second and fourth quarters. So, in a 30-minute game with 10 players, each player would play 15 minutes.

If you have eight players for a 30-minute game, each player would get close to 19 minutes of playing time, if they got equal time. When your number of players doesn't divide evenly into the number of minutes, it makes it more difficult to give everyone equal time, but the point here is if you are coaching 6- to 8-year-olds, don't forget about one or two of your least-talented kids. Get them in the game because that's what they're there for.

For ages nine and above, you might begin to dole out minutes based more on skill, though you still want to play all your players. Look to get your lesser-talented players in for a decent amount of time.

note

Be aware of your league rules regarding substitutions. Most leagues allow substitutions only during stops in the game, but some leagues allow substitutions to be made "on the fly," with a player entering and another leaving as the game is going on.

Appropriate Behavior

Remember that all eyes are upon you, at one time or another, during a game. Of most importance are the eyes of your players. They see how you behave, and that greatly impacts how they behave, or at least how they think they should behave.

Be positive, be encouraging, and cheer your team on. If you want to discuss a play with a referee, do so respectfully and without making a big show of it.

Coach your players to be good sports, and lead the way by being one yourself. Don't argue with opposing coaches, don't say derogatory things to opposing players, and don't root *against* the opposing team. Simply root *for* your team.

Coach your players to play hard, to play fair, and to play to win. Let your players know in advance how you will respond if they do or say something unsporting at a game, and follow through. For a mild infraction of your rules, talk to them, correct them, and give them one more chance. For a second mild infraction, take them out of the game. For a major infraction, even if it's the first, take them out of the game. In either case, consider suspending them for another game if you believe the infraction warrants such a response.

Sports offer an arena for kids to not only practice their physical skills, but also learn discipline, the proper expression of emotion, patience, and respect for themselves and others. And the person they learn most from is you.

After the Game

After the game, line your players up for a team handshake with their opponents. (Instruct your players in practice how you want them to behave during this post-game handshake.) Have them shake or slap hands and offer "Good game" or some similar comment to their opponents. Be clear with your players that you want them to refrain from saying anything derogatory, no matter what happened during the game. The team handshake is an important part of youth sports because it teaches respect for the opponent and helps keep the contest in perspective.

If you win, celebrate, but do so in a manner that doesn't rub it in to the other team. If you lose, don't hang your heads. Either way, go through the team handshake, thank the referees for taking their time to officiate the game, and then hold a brief post-game meeting.

Team Meeting

Hold a brief meeting before letting the kids go. This isn't the time to go into great detail, but let them know what they did well, what they still need to work on, and give them some positives to take home. Note areas where they have improved, note plays or situations in which they performed well, and help them keep the outcome in perspective. Help them learn from the game, whether they won or lost. For some thoughts on what you can learn from winning and losing, see the following sidebar, "Lessons of the Game."

Finally, remind your players of the next practice or game, and make sure they all have rides before you leave the gym. Don't leave a child waiting for a ride, even if he says he's waiting to be picked up by a parent; make sure he gets his ride before you leave.

LESSONS OF THE GAME

What can players learn from a win? They can learn that

- Hard effort sometimes pays off. So maybe all that time spent in practice is worth it after all!

- Sometimes you're better than the other team, and it shows. But don't rest on your laurels because another game is coming.

- Sometimes you get lucky. The best team doesn't always win, and your team can win on any given day.

- Winning is a team effort. Contributions to a win can come from unexpected places.

A win feels great, so celebrate. But remember the following:

- A win is good for only one game. Don't get too cocky.
- You don't have to be perfect to win. Don't get down on yourself for a missed shot or a turnover.
- A game's not over until no time is left on the clock. Never think you can coast home to victory.
- Basketball is a game in which you can redeem yourself. Your final shot can erase that earlier turnover you made.

Basketball is a game through which players can learn about respect, hard work, teamwork, patience, persistence, and much more. It's also a game that teaches through defeat. Losses are never fun, but through a loss, players can learn the following:

- Sometimes you're better than the other team, and you still lose.
- Sometimes the other team is simply better than you.
- Sometimes you just have an off day, or you get unlucky.
- Sometimes you can work really hard and still lose.

Losing doesn't feel so hot. But remember the following:

- A loss is only for one game. Don't get too down.
- Pride comes before a fall. Don't chalk up a win before you take to the court.
- A game's not over until the clock reads 0:00. Never give up.

The Absolute Minimum

This chapter helped you consider all the issues involved in coaching during games. Among the key points were

- At the practice before the game, go over the game particulars—the gym location, the time you want players to arrive, and so forth—and the game plan.
- Keep your tactics simple, especially at younger levels.
- Base your game plan and tactics on your team's strengths and abilities and on the opponent's weaknesses.
- Save the pregame speech. Just help your players focus on the fundamentals and game plan.

continues

■ Be aware of the signs of over- and under-coaching and steer toward a happy medium, being involved and encouraging but not directing your players' every move.

■ Give your players guidance and technique tips, but don't overload them with information or corrections during games.

■ Consider playing time issues and plan to give your players appropriate time on the court.

■ Display appropriate behavior at games. Remember that you are your players' role model.

■ Lead your team in post-game handshakes with the opponents and hold a brief meeting afterward. Help your players take home positives from the game, regardless of the outcome.

■ Help your players learn from both wins and losses.

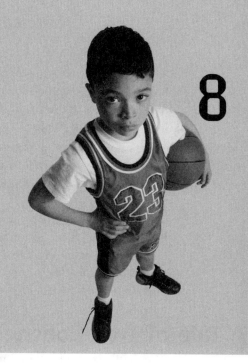

8

Ingredients of a Successful Season

The final game of the season is over and your players shake hands with the opponents. You hold a brief team meeting, and afterward, as most of the other team's players depart, many of your players hang around with their parents or friends, joking, shooting baskets, and having fun. Four of your players begin an impromptu 2-on-2 game, and one player makes a great cut, receives a pass, and scores.

You can't help but smile. "Hey, you goofballs!" you call out to the four who are playing. "You should have done a little more of that this season!"

To a casual observer, it would be hard to tell that your team had just lost its final game and finished with a 3-9 record. That casual observer might think, from the way your team is carrying on, that you just won the league championship.

You didn't, at least numbers-wise. You finished in the lower half of the pack. But basketball, even with all its statistics, is so much more than numbers. And, for that matter, success at the youth level is so much more than winning percentages, league titles, and trophies.

There's nothing wrong, of course, with winning the league title or having a good winning percentage. In fact, that's what every team strives for. Those just aren't the only indicators of success, and you need to measure your accomplishments as a coach in other ways.

Why? There are many answers to that question, but two will suffice here. First, the hand you were dealt, in terms of player talent, doesn't always come up aces. Sometimes it comes up a mixture of low, unmatched cards. Second, the winning percentage or league trophy simply doesn't tell the complete story. Consider the following two cases.

A Tale of Two Coaches

The Celtics compiled a 10-2 regular season record and went on to win the Border League championship. Yet, after the title game, the players' celebration was strangely subdued, showing as much relief as joy. Coach Taylor didn't take part in the celebration, but watched it with an air of satisfaction and pride. No player came over to congratulate Coach Taylor, and he made no move to congratulate any player.

At a players-only pizza party that night, the conversation went like this:

"I'm glad that's over."

"Me too. I couldn't wait."

"I wonder what Coach Taylor would have said if we lost?"

"Probably what he said after our two regular season losses, only ten times worse."

"I'm not playing next year."

"Me either."

"Why not?"

"Are you kidding? You want to go through that again?"

Coach Taylor got the most out of his players' ability. He knew the game, he knew the skills and how to teach them, and he prepared his players to compete.

But he also trampled all over them emotionally and psychologically. Three players played the absolute minimum the league would allow. He yelled at players for making mistakes, the veins sticking out in his neck as he did, and he made players run laps and do pushups for every turnover they made. He cried out in disgust when they missed shots in key situations. He berated the referees; no one liked to referee the Celtics' games.

No one caught him smiling all season long. His normal pose was standing by the bench, scowling, his arms folded across his thick chest, a critical look in his eye. He shouted harshly enough at four players to make them cry, and when they cried, he ridiculed them for being babies.

The Pacers, on the other hand, finished the regular season at 4-8 and got knocked out of the playoffs in the first round, losing 28-24 to the Celtics. (After that game, Coach Taylor spent 10 minutes lambasting his players for almost getting beat by "a bunch of pansies" and told his players they might as well go home and play with their dolls if they couldn't play any better than that.)

The Pacers were disappointed that they were beaten, but they had a festive pizza party afterward, and the players presented Coach Giles with a "Coach of the Year" plaque.

Coach of the Year for a 4-8 team? Though it was not an official league award, it well could have been. Consider these items:

- All of Coach Giles's players were as happy and excited about basketball at the end of the season as they were at the beginning.
- All his players improved their skills throughout the season.
- They also gained in their understanding of the game's tactics and rules.
- The Pacers played hard every game, getting the most out of their abilities. They never gave up, and they didn't mope after losses.
- They pulled together as a team, rooting each other on, enjoying each other's successes, and encouraging each other after a failed attempt.
- The Pacers *did* win an official league title—the sporting behavior award as "Best Sports."
- Everyone played, everyone improved, and everyone had fun.

Of course, many championship teams are coached very well and are successful not only in their win-loss record, but also in the ways the Pacers were successful. That wasn't the case with the Celtics and Coach Taylor, however.

Which coach would *you* rather be: Coach Taylor or Coach Giles?

Evaluating Your Season

If winning isn't the only way to evaluate your success, what are the measures you should use? What are the keys to having a truly successful season? Throughout the rest of this chapter we focus on those keys. They shouldn't come as a surprise to you because they're a summation of everything you've learned in the first seven chapters.

These same keys provide the foundation for Appendix F, "Season Evaluation Form." After you read this chapter and complete your season, use Appendix F to evaluate your own season.

Did Your Players Have Fun?

As you'll recall from Chapter 1, "Your Coaching Approach," having fun is the main reason kids play basketball. That's an easy enough concept for most coaches to grasp before the season begins, but after the practices get underway, that concept can get lost amidst the more immediate and pressing goals and duties of a coach.

Can you win without having fun? Yes. But consider this: By the time kids reach age 13, their drop-out rate from sports is 75%. Some of that attrition is due to simply a lack of ability to compete at their age level anymore. Some of it is due to new interests that take up their time, such as music, art, or drama. But for the most part, players drop out of sports because

- They don't get enough playing time. Consistently when asked, kids respond they'd rather play for a losing team than sit on the bench for a winning team.
- They don't learn the skills they need to be competitive.
- They feel like failures (mainly because they haven't learned the skills). Their coaches don't reinforce their competence or help them see the positive aspects of their performance.
- They receive too much negative feedback from coaches.
- The sports environment is too negative; it's not enjoyable to go to practices or games.
- They stress out over winning because winning is overemphasized.
- Practices are poorly organized, tedious, and boring. Drills are repetitive, players are inactive, and the fun is drained out of the experience.

"Fun," then, doesn't mean telling jokes at practice, or goofing off, or trying to entertain your players. It means giving them playing time and building their skills so they'll feel competent when they have that playing time. It means reinforcing the skills they have and helping them focus on their positives, rather than dwelling on their negatives. It means giving them feedback but couching it in positive terms. It means making practices active, meaningful, and enjoyable, using a variety of games and drills that are game-like and that help them build their skills.

What are indications that your players are having fun? It's easy to see in the smiles on their faces, their body language, their focus, their effort, and their encouragement of each other.

Perhaps the greatest indication of all, though, is that they're happy at the end of the season no matter what their record was, and they can't wait for next basketball season to roll around.

Did Your Players Learn New Skills and Improve on Previously Learned Skills?

In considering player performances, all too often a season is judged on where the players ended, without regard to where they *began*. The true measure of success here is how much your players improved over the season. If they were good to begin with and ended up being good, without showing any real improvement, something went wrong. If they were poor to begin with and ended up being average, that's showing improvement.

Here are some of the mistakes coaches make in this area:

- They lack the teaching skills or technical know-how to help their players learn new skills or improve ones they've already learned.

- They are poor practice planners, meaning they squander their practice time or run ineffective drills.

- They push players to learn too fast or present advanced skills and tactics too early.

- They don't present advanced skills and tactics as the players develop; they keep them at an elementary level and don't help them hone skills.

- They focus on their better players and offer little help to their lesser-skilled players.

The best coaches can work with kids of varying abilities and help them all progress. They don't ignore their lesser-skilled players, and they adjust their teaching plan according to the skill levels of the kids, always gently pushing for improvement.

To foster such improvement, first you need to be able to plan and conduct effective practices. You also need a critical eye to assess talent and needs, the teaching skills to instruct and reinforce your players on the correct techniques, plenty of patience because players seem to sometimes take one step forward and two steps backward in learning, and the ability to encourage and support your players as they continue their growth.

note

There's great joy as a coach in watching good players perform up to their capabilities. There's also great joy in helping lesser-talented players pick up skills and perform beyond where they or anyone else thought they were capable of performing.

Every season is a building season, an opportunity for players to become better, build on their talent and success, and come back for an even better year next year because they have deepened and broadened their abilities.

Did You Help Your Players Understand the Game and Its Rules?

Lots of games are decided by players' physical skills—by their abilities to shoot, pass, dribble, rebound, and play defense.

And a lot of games are decided by players' abilities to apply the rules and execute the strategies: Alex keeps camping out in the lane and several offensive rebounds and second-chance baskets are lost because he's called for three-second violations. Darnell doesn't realize you can't be moving when you set a screen and a crucial basket late in the game is wiped out because he committed a foul while setting a screen. Abbie forgets that you can't dribble again after you've picked up your dribble, and commits a turnover that leads to the game-winning basket for the other team. The list could go on and on.

It's tempting to focus solely on teaching skills because that's such an obvious need. But players, especially at the youth level, need to also grasp the bigger picture of how to perform those skills and how to use their abilities within the rules to benefit their team. They need to understand the "when" as well as the "how" of performing skills.

When you build the teaching of rules and strategies into your drills and practice games, you are one step ahead of most coaches—and one step closer to building a competitive, savvy squad that knows how to play the game and does the little things that help to win games.

Did You Communicate Appropriately and Effectively?

Basketball courts across America are filled with coaches who don't know how to communicate well. Why? Because they think their ability to talk qualifies them as good communicators. (Of course, having read Chapter 3, "Communication Keys," you know this is far from the truth.)

Some of the signs of poor and ineffective communication include

- Players don't learn skills because the coach can't communicate clearly.
- Parents aren't kept informed and don't know how to pitch in and help.
- Players hang their heads or begin to miss practices because their coach yells at, degrades, or berates them.
- Players look bored or confused because their coach uses 100 words when 10 would suffice.

■ Players don't listen to their coach because he doesn't speak with command or authority. This has nothing to do with volume or gruffness; it has everything to do with understanding, preparation, clarity, and delivery.

■ Players aren't sure what to do in certain game situations because their coach hasn't told them.

■ Players don't pay attention because their coach doesn't know how to get and hold their attention.

■ Players appear wary and unsure because their coach said one thing but her body language said something different.

■ Messages get lost, feelings get hurt, and sometimes tempers flare because the coach is too busy talking to listen to players or parents.

■ Players, parents, and coaches become frustrated.

Your ability to communicate has significant impact on your overall coaching effectiveness. As you teach skills, do you clearly demonstrate them and use language your players can understand? As you correct mistakes and encourage players, what does your body language communicate, and is it in sync with your words? Do you *listen* to your players' comments and questions, and do you read and interpret their body language, as surely as they do yours?

Did you communicate with parents before the season, letting them know your philosophy and coaching approach, your expectations of the players, and what the players and parents could expect of you? Are you maintaining a healthy flow of communication with parents as the season progresses?

note

Do you maintain control of your emotions as you communicate? Note that this doesn't mean you don't *show* emotion; it means you *control* it.

Did You Provide for Your Players' Safety?

Providing for your players' safety doesn't mean no injuries happen on your watch. It means, ideally, that no *preventable* injuries happen and that whatever injuries *do* happen, you tend to them appropriately.

It's all in the planning and preparation. You plan for safety, you take the necessary precautions, and (when need be) you respond to the abrasion, bump, bruise, or twisted ankle when it occurs.

You are on your way to fulfilling your responsibilities here if you

■ Are trained in CPR and first aid

■ Have a well-stocked first aid kit on hand at practices and games, and know how to use it

- Make sure you know of any allergies or medical conditions of players, and know how to respond if the allergies or conditions flare up
- Warn your players and their parents of the inherent risks of basketball
- Check the practice and game courts for safety hazards and eliminate those hazards, if possible, before playing on the courts
- Enforce rules regarding player behavior that enhance player safety
- Provide proper supervision throughout each practice
- Offer proper skill instruction
- Take a water break during practice

Did You Plan and Conduct Effective Practices?

If you played youth sports, you undoubtedly attended a practice or two in which your coach was winging it. His "preparation" time was spent driving to the gym, and the drills he chose seemed to have no real purpose to them, other than to bore you to tears. You didn't learn any new skills or refine the ones you had; you simply spent time—and poorly, at that.

Have you spent time planning your season and your practices? Are you effective in running your practices? Signs of effectiveness include

- Kids pay attention to you because you have a purpose to what you're doing.
- There is no down time while you're trying to figure out what to do next.
- Players are active and engaged; they aren't standing around waiting for a turn. You use multiple stations when appropriate.
- You use games and drills that are designed to teach a specific skill or tactic you want your players to work on that day.
- Your players are learning new skills and refining ones they have.
- Your players are having fun in practice.

There's one more sign you're planning and conducting well: *you're* having fun, too. When you're prepared and your practices have a purpose to them, it's enjoyable for everyone involved.

Did Your Players Give Maximum Effort in Practices and Games?

You might wonder why this question would be part of evaluating your success. After all, motivation comes from within; you can't make your kids try harder.

This is true. But you can create an environment that increases the likelihood your players will give full effort. Conversely, you can create an environment that stifles motivation.

Obviously, you want to do the former and not the latter. Before detailing the type of environment that motivates kids, let's consider the type of environment that leaves them high and dry.

Some of the ways a coach can demotivate players include

- Yelling at them for mistakes and for their general quality of play
- Comparing a child to a better player
- Having kids wait in line to take their turn
- Not teaching players the skills they need
- Appearing to not care about their performances or about them as individuals
- Playing favorites, and paying little attention to lesser-talented children
- Not listening to them

Some coaches mistakenly believe yelling is the best motivator. Their players do become motivated to behave in a way that makes their coach stop yelling, which, it might be argued, is the coach's point. But if you yell at a kid to catch the ball before he looks to shoot or pass or dribble, using an angry or irritated tone of voice, the child will often respond by becoming tense and anxious, which increases the likelihood that he'll drop the next pass thrown to him.

Is it wrong to tell the player to catch the ball? Not at all. It's wrong to yell it at him, showing your anger or irritation.

So, how do you create an environment in which your players are motivated to do their best? You do so by

- Teaching players the skills they need
- Giving kids specific technique goals to work toward
- Giving specific, positive feedback as players work on their skills
- Encouraging kids, especially when they get down, and praising correct technique and effort
- Helping kids take home the positives of the practice or game
- Praising hustle, desire, and teamwork shown in practice and games
- Running efficient, purposeful practices in which players are active and engaged the whole time

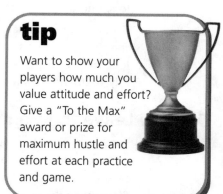

tip

Want to show your players how much you value attitude and effort? Give a "To the Max" award or prize for maximum hustle and effort at each practice and game.

■ Valuing each child for his or her own abilities and personality

■ Caring about the kids as players and as children

■ Listening to players

When you create an environment in which your players are motivated to learn and perform, you'll reap the rewards in practices and games.

Did Your Players Leave the Games on the Court?

League games can be highly emotional events. The players are performing in front of parents, other family members, and their peers. They want to play well. They want to win. Some of them have dreams of becoming an NBA player some day.

Then a pass goes right through their hands. They miss an easy layup. They commit two turnovers in a row. They commit fouls that they normally never commit. They mount a comeback, only to fall short by one point.

Individual failures and team losses are not easy to take, but all players have to learn how to deal with personal and team setbacks. Losing happens. In fact, it happens once a game. Kids have widely divergent reactions to losing. Often, at younger ages, you can't tell which team won by the responses and behaviors of both teams immediately following the game. Sometimes, though, defeats can have an impact on kids, no matter what age they are.

Realize that while they take many cues from you, they also are heavily influenced by their parents' views on winning and losing and by the cultural stigma attached to losing. Some kids take losing very personally; some feel it marks them somehow; some feel they let their teammates down; some respond by being poor sports; others don't know how to master the emotions that come with disappointment.

Part of your duty is to help them master those emotions, keep the game in perspective, and leave it (whether it was a win or a loss) on the court. They can't erase a loss, and they can't carry forward a win. They start out 0-0 in their next game.

Talk to your team before the first game about keeping the wins and losses in perspective, and then watch for players who are too high after a win or too low after a loss. Help your players keep a level head if they win a big game or play exceptionally well, and help them look forward to the next game if they lose or play poorly.

Did *You* Leave the Games on the Court?

Jerry was coaxed to coach the Lakers, his son Brandon's team, at the last minute. He went into the season with much trepidation because he had never coached before. But he found he liked it, and he had a good team and they played well—"in spite of the coaching they get," Jerry wryly told his friends.

They won their first three games, including an upset against the Pistons, the league's best team from the previous year. The Pistons had most of their players back.

The next game, though, the Lakers lost to the Hornets, who weren't all that good. To his chagrin and surprise, Jerry didn't sleep very well that night. He couldn't believe he could lose sleep over a youth basketball game. But he did.

As the season went on, the Lakers and the Pistons were running neck and neck for first place. They each accumulated three losses in the regular season, and Jerry took each loss harder than the previous loss.

"It's all right, Dad," Brandon told his dad on the way home after the Lakers' second loss.

After the third loss, Brandon said nothing on the way home because his dad was too upset. "There's no way we should have lost to the Knicks!" Jerry groused to no one in particular as he drove home. "That referee called it one way for the Knicks, and another way for us. It was ridiculous."

That might have been true, but what was *more* ridiculous was Jerry's response to the loss. He not only didn't leave the game at the court, but also took it home with him, slept with it, and got up the next morning and dragged it to work with him.

It's easy to get wrapped up in the wins and losses, to care so much about the kids and want them to win so badly that you let the game's outcome affect you more than it should. Care about the outcome, yes. By all means care about the kids. But do what you want them to do: Leave it at the gym and come prepared to the next practice to go forward, leaving behind any baggage from the last game.

Did You Conduct Yourself Appropriately?

As you know, you're a role model for your players. How good a model you are is up to you. A few signs of a good role model include

- You communicate in positive ways with opposing coaches and players and with referees.
- You coach within the rules and have your players play within them.
- You maintain control of your emotions in practices and games while providing the coaching and support your players need.
- You keep the games in perspective and help your players do the same.

Remember this: Briefly losing your cool does not necessarily mean you failed as a role model. In fact, you can use such an instance to send a healthy message to your players. When you admit that you made a mistake and apologize for it, you set a positive example for the kids.

Did You Communicate Effectively with Parents and Involve Them in Positive Ways?

Some coaches put up with parents. Others look to placate them and hold them at bay. Still others do their best to ignore them, communicating with them as little as possible.

These coaches are missing the boat. At worst they are inviting trouble, and at the least they are overlooking a rich source of support and help.

Parents are your chief allies, and most parents want to help in some way, to make the sport experience as good as possible for their son or daughter. Yes, there are parents who present problems to coaches, but these are in the minority.

You read in Chapter 3 about ways to communicate with and involve parents. If you have healthy communication and involvement throughout the season, it probably looks something like this:

- You have few or no misunderstandings with parents regarding your coaching philosophy.
- You delegate responsibilities, sharing the workload with a lot of parents—and making your program stronger in doing so.
- You aren't as stressed as you might be, had you not involved parents.
- You appropriately address the few misunderstandings or concerns parents have.

When you have a good communication flow with parents and involve them in your program, everyone benefits.

Did You Coach Appropriately During Games?

Some coaches don't make the distinction between coaching in practices and coaching at games, and their players suffer for it. In Chapter 7, "Game Time!" you learned of the perils of over-coaching and under-coaching and the keys of effective coaching during games.

So, what does effective coaching during games look like? You get high marks for game-day coaching if most of these statements apply to your game days:

- You keep your strategy simple and base it on your players' strengths and abilities and on your opponent's weaknesses.
- You help your players get mentally prepared for the game by focusing them on the fundamentals they need to execute and on the game plan.
- You provide tactical direction and guidance throughout the game.
- You are encouraging and supportive.
- You give technique tips and reminders, and let the kids play, saving the mistake correction for the next practice.

- You tend to the kids' needs during the game—emotional and psychological as well as mental and physical.
- You help players keep the game in proper perspective.
- You use a positive coaching approach.
- You effectively rotate players in and out.
- Your players conduct themselves well during and after the game, including the post-game handshake.
- You hold a brief post-game meeting, giving the kids some positives to take home, regardless of the outcome of the game.

Coach games in a manner that helps kids develop their skills, learn the game, compete well, and enjoy the experience. When you do that, you're assured of a winning season, no matter what your record is.

Did You Win with Class and Lose with Dignity?

Many players learn how to shoot, pass, dribble, rebound, and play defense. Plenty of players enjoy good seasons, and numerous teams enjoy superlative winning records.

Unfortunately, not all those players and teams learn how to handle their successes. Puffed up with their own accomplishments, they taunt or trash talk the other team during the game and celebrate the victory after the game in a way that rubs the loss in to the other team.

Your coaching duties don't end with teaching your team how to execute and how to compete and win. It extends to teaching them how to handle victories and defeats.

Winning and losing are part of life, and the lessons the players can learn through basketball can help them deal with wins and losses in other arenas throughout their lives.

Here's what winning with class looks like:

- You and your players shake hands with the other team, offering them congratulations.
- You thank the referees for volunteering their time.
- Your team celebrates fully but in a way that shows respect for the other team.

And here's what losing with dignity looks like:

- Your players don't hang their heads, no matter how hard the loss was.
- You and your players congratulate the other team, looking them in the eye as you do.

■ You thank the referees for volunteering their time.

■ You hold a brief team meeting and help the players regroup and take home positives from the game.

The ability to be gracious in victory and disappointed yet not defeated when you're on the short end of the score is all about character. You can help your players build character throughout the season, not only in games but in practices as well. Players can build character by having respect for themselves and others, by caring for others, by maintaining their integrity and by following through on their responsibilities.

note

Kids can give their all on the court, but they can't control the outcome of the game. When you help your players build character, they will know how to win with class and lose with dignity.

Did You Make the Experience Positive, Meaningful, and Fun for Your Players?

This is what it all boils down to: Was the experience positive for your players? Was it fun? Did it leave them wanting to come back for more? Championships or winning records don't mean much if the players can't wait for the season to end and half of them don't return the next year for a repeat performance.

Was the season meaningful to your players? Did they learn the skills and tactics, the game, and the rules? Did they learn about themselves, how they respond to challenges, how to win, how to lose? Did they build character? For some telltale signs of a season that was positive, meaningful, and fun, see the following sidebar, "Signs of a Season Well Spent."

If your players show at the end of the season the same zest and enthusiasm that they showed at the beginning, you know you did well in this area. And you can look forward to welcoming them back next season.

SIGNS OF A SEASON WELL SPENT

Here are some signs of a memorable season. Hopefully, you will be able to identify with some of these signs when your season concludes:

■ "Yeah, we were 5-7. We lost a couple of tough games, and we had a few games where we didn't play so well. But you know what? The kids improved over the season. They were really clicking and playing well at the end. And they had fun through it all." —*Coach Williams*

■ "Cody was the worst player on our team throughout most of the season. He didn't even want the ball passed to him in the beginning. But he really blossomed at the end; he somehow gained the confidence to get in there and play, and he never gave up on himself. His fundamentals improved dramatically from beginning to end. You should have seen the smile on his face when he made some good passes and hit a few shots! I had lots of kids who played better, but I was happiest of all for Cody." —*Coach Yarborough*

- "I'd say, 'Molly, do you understand that reaching in and contacting the player with the ball is a foul?' and she'd say, 'Yes.' Then she'd reach in and foul the next time down the court. I'd say, 'Molly, remember, you can't reach in.' And she'd say, 'Okay.' And she'd reach in the next time, too. It took her half the season to get it. But she finally got it. I thought her teammates were going to lift her on their shoulders when she stopped reaching in!" —*Coach Mancini*

- "I just want to thank you for working so patiently with Andre. I know he gets distracted and he sometimes doesn't listen, or he forgets. Your patience made a big difference—and it showed in his play." —*Andre's mother*

- "I was really impressed with your practices; the team Jeremy was on last year wasn't run nearly so well. Jeremy learned so much more this year. Thanks, too, for letting me get involved. I really enjoyed helping you out." —*Jeremy's father*

- "Thanks for being a good role model for DeShawn. He's so competitive and he *hates* to lose. It's easy for his temper to get the best of him. The way you kept your cool during games really showed him something. Every time he wanted to blame a referee or complain about the other team, you focused his attention on his own performance. I think he really grew up this season. Thank you!" —*DeShawn's mother*

- "Hey, Coach, is there a spring league?" —*Your players*

THE ABSOLUTE MINIMUM

This chapter focused on the ingredients of a successful season. That success can be evidenced in a good win-loss record, but that just scratches the surface. Digging a little deeper, true success in a basketball season is evidenced by these signs:

- Your players learned the skills, tactics, and rules they needed to know to compete to the best of their abilities.

- Your players were mentally, emotionally, and physically ready to play each game.

- Your players improved their skills and understanding of the game over the season.

- Your players had fun at practices and games.

- Your players displayed good sporting behavior throughout the season.

- You communicated appropriately with everyone involved—players, parents, referees, and league administrators—and involved parents in your program.

continues

- You planned and conducted practices effectively, keeping players actively engaged and presenting skills in a logical order.
- You taught skills and tactics effectively, showing and demonstrating how they should be performed and putting kids in game-like situations to practice the tactics and skills.
- Your players gave maximum effort in practices and games.
- You provided the coaching the kids needed during the games.
- You and your players gave each game your best and, win or lose, you all were able to leave the game on the court and keep the outcome in perspective.
- You taught your players to win with class and lose with dignity and guided them in doing so, leading by example.

PART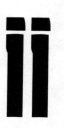

Sᴋɪʟʟs ᴀɴᴅ Tᴀᴄᴛɪᴄs

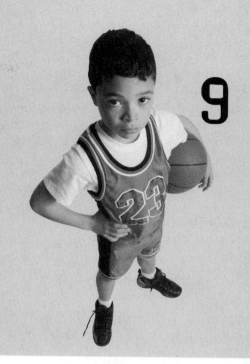

9

OFFENSIVE SKILLS AND TACTICS

In Chapter 5, "Practice Plans," you learned about planning your season and your individual practices, and in Chapter 6, "Player Development," you learned the method of teaching skills. Now, in the next two chapters, you'll be presented with the mechanics for all the skills and tactics you'll need to teach. Then, in Chapter 11, "Games and Drills," you'll find games and drills you can use to teach the skills and tactics.

In this chapter, the focus is on dribbling, passing, shooting, rebounding, and other offensive skills and tactics. Use this chapter to learn about the proper execution of offensive skills and tactics and to refresh your memory before you teach the skills and tactics to your players.

Triple-threat Stance

From a triple-threat stance, a player can shoot, dribble, or pass. Upon receiving the ball, and before dribbling, the player places his weight forward on the balls of his feet and holds the ball at chest level, elbows out (see Figure 9.1). He is bent at the waist and knees and can drive or pass in any direction, or fake a move and then draw back and shoot.

Footwork

Footwork skills are among the most important skills you can teach your players. The ability to use their feet well can gain them an advantage in a variety of situations. On the flip side, if they don't develop good footwork skills, they will be called for traveling and miss out on opportunities to gain some space between themselves and their defender.

Teach your players how to perform pivots, cuts, jump stops, stride stops, jab steps, and rocker steps.

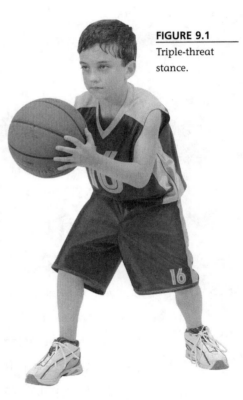

FIGURE 9.1
Triple-threat
stance.

Pivot

If a player moves both her feet while holding the ball and not dribbling, she will be called for traveling. She can, however, freely move one foot in any direction while keeping a *pivot foot* in the same place on the court (see Figure 9.2).
She can pick the heel of her pivot foot off the ground and swivel on that foot, so long as the toes remain in the same place on the court.

After she moves one foot, the other foot must remain in contact with the court as the pivot foot. After stopping her dribble, she cannot pick up her pivot foot and touch it down again before she releases the ball. Likewise, if she has caught a pass, she can pivot on one foot before dribbling.

Pivoting is an important skill because it allows a player to move her body to protect the ball from a defender. It can also help a player get in better position to shoot.

FIGURE 9.2

Pivoting on one foot.

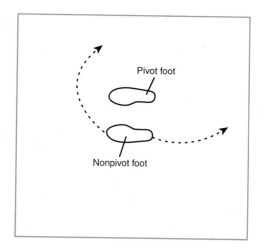

Cut

Players *cut* to change direction. By making sharp cuts, they can gain a step or two on their defender. They can make cuts while dribbling, or without the ball, to get open for a pass or to get in better position to rebound.

Teach players to push hard off one foot to change their direction. The crisper and sharper the cut, the greater the advantage, as long as they maintain control of their bodies.

Players can use cuts to get open anywhere on the court. A particularly effective type of cut is the *backdoor cut* (see Figure 9.3), in which a player moves away from the basket, and then cuts toward it. This type of cut is usually made when the defender gets off balance or when the attacker sees his defender glance at the basketball. Teach your players to get a hand up and to look for the ball as they make their cut. The advantage gained in making the cut will be negated if they aren't ready to catch the pass.

Jump Stop

A player executes a *jump stop* by using both feet to come to a stop. A jump stop is used after catching a pass while on the move. It helps the player gain control of his body. In such a stop, both feet hit the floor at the same time. After the stop, the player can use either foot for a pivot.

Stride Stop

A player can use a *stride stop* to shoot off the dribble. As a right-handed player picks up his dribble, he steps forward with his left foot, hitting on his heel to help him stop. He strides forward with his right foot, bending his knees and keeping his feet shoulder-width apart, ready to shoot (see Figure 9.4).

FIGURE 9.3
Backdoor cut.

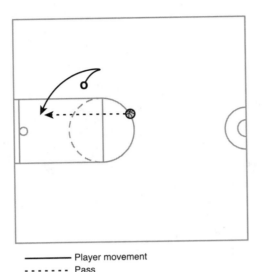

————— Player movement
- - - - - - Pass

FIGURE 9.4
(a) The player
steps forward
with his left foot.
(b) He then
strides with his
right foot and
prepares to shoot
or pass.

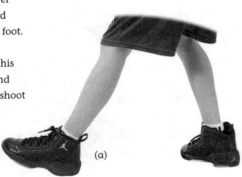
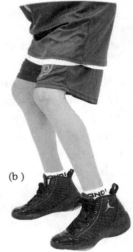

(b)

(a)

Jab Step

A *jab step* is a short, quick step used by a player with the ball to fake her opponent. The player takes a quick step forward with her nonpivot foot, and then draws it quickly back. Such a move opens up space between the player with the ball and the defender. An effective jab step generally causes the defender to back up to guard against a drive to the basket. This step is most useful when the player is in shooting range, to open up a shooting opportunity.

note

To be effective, a jab step must be taken in a way that makes the defender think the player is going to try to dribble past the defender. The step must be hard, quick, and directly toward the defender, slightly outside the defender's back foot.

Rocker Step

A player can use a *rocker step*, which is a quick head-and-shoulder fake, to set up a drive or a shot. To execute a rocker step, the player keeps the ball at waist level, takes a short, quick step toward the defender, fakes a dribble by bringing the ball down outside the knee, and then rocks back to his original position. If the defender takes a step back to defend against the drive, the player is open for a shot. If the defender moves up to closely guard the ball handler, the player can use a powerful step and strong dribble past the hip of his defender. See Figure 9.5 for an illustration of the rocker step.

FIGURE 9.5

(a) The player begins with the ball at waist level. (b) After taking a quick step toward the defender and faking a dribble, he rocks back.

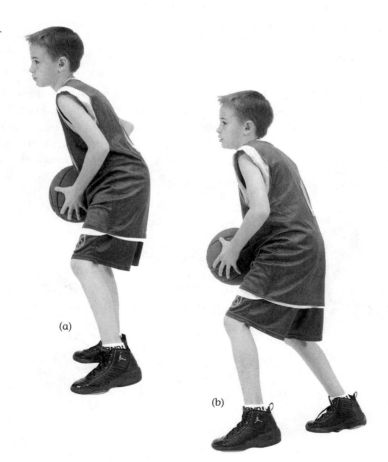

(a)

(b)

Dribbling

Dribbling—that is, bouncing the ball on the floor—is one way to advance the ball. If the player with the ball wants to advance it while maintaining possession of the ball, he has to dribble it; otherwise, he'll be called for traveling.

There are several types of dribbles you can teach your players, including control, speed, crossover, spin, and half-spin dribbles. For younger players, just focus on the control dribble. As they master the control dribble, teach them the speed dribble. Older and more skilled players can learn the other dribbles.

Control Dribble

In teaching control dribbling, focus on these five aspects:

- **Use the fingertips, not the palm, to control the ball**—If players use their palms to dribble, they have no control.

- **Develop your strong hand first, and then learn to dribble with your "weak" hand**—Certainly players should practice with their strong hand first, but after they have the basics down with that hand, they should also develop their skills with their other hand. Being able to dribble with both hands will help players maintain possession and be more of a threat.

- **Keep the ball low as you dribble, and maintain good athletic position**—A common mistake young dribblers make is to bounce the ball too high. This makes it easier for a defender to steal the ball. Teach your players to dribble waist height or lower and to be in an athletic position, with knees and waist bent, to help them stay low and thus present less of a target for their defender (see Figure 9.6).

FIGURE 9.6
Keeping the ball low, maintaining good position, and shielding the ball from the defender. Notice the dribbler's head is up to see the court.

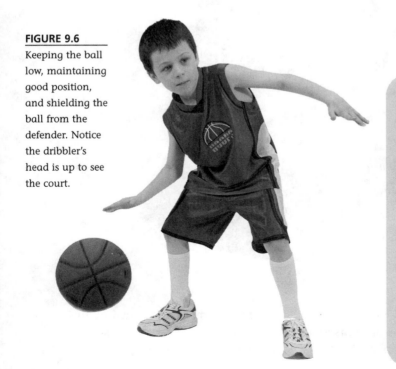

note

Players tend to dribble too much. Dribbling is an essential skill to learn, and an appropriate way to move the ball up the court and to drive toward the basket, but teach your players to be looking to pass, and to pass whenever it gains them an advantage. Why? They can move the ball faster by passing than by dribbling, and it's usually easier to defend against dribbling than against passing.

- **Protect the ball as you dribble**—Players need to learn how to protect the ball as they dribble—how to use their bodies to shield the ball from the player guarding them (see Figure 9.6).

- **Keep your head up so you can see the court**—Another common error players make is to watch the ball as they dribble. This makes it easier for the defense to steal the ball, and it also results in missed opportunities because the dribbler can't see open teammates.

Speed Dribble

A player uses the *speed dribble* when she's in open court, such as after a steal or on a fast break. After players learn the basics of dribbling, they can practice speed dribbling.

Unlike control dribbling, the player isn't trying to keep the ball close to her on the speed dribble. She can push it out in front of her, allowing her to run after it, and she should keep it at about waist height. The object is to go as fast as possible while maintaining control of the ball.

The player's hand is not directly over the ball, but is behind it at about a 45° angle as she pushes it out in front of her. She completely extends her arm as she continues to push the ball out in front.

Crossover Dribble

A skilled dribbler can use a *crossover dribble* when his defender is overplaying his strong side. To execute a crossover, the dribbler needs to be able to dribble well with either hand. For a right-handed player to execute a crossover dribble when he is overplayed on his right side, he should

1. Make a jab step in the direction of the defensive player with the right foot.
2. Take a long step with the right foot, crossing it over the outside of the defender's right foot.
3. Swing the ball quickly from his right side to his left side, cutting closely by the defender's shoulder.
4. Push the ball out past the defender's hip with his left hand.

See Figure 9.7 for a crossover dribble.

FIGURE 9.7
(a) To begin a crossover dribble, the player takes a jab step. (b) He steps over the defender's foot and crosses the ball over. (c) He dribbles past the defender, using the opposite hand.

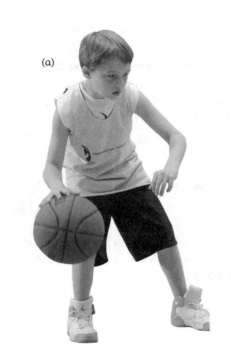

(a)

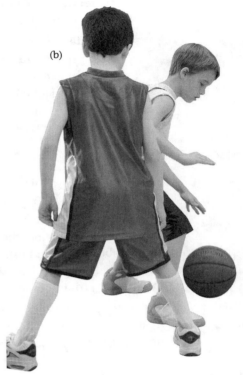

(b)

(c)

Spin Dribble

A player can use a *spin dribble* to elude a defender when he is closely guarded. The player dribbles in one direction, and then quickly stops, reverse pivots, and pulls the ball behind him as he spins. At the end of the spin, he switches hands and explodes past the defender. The dribbler should keep his dribble low while executing the spin dribble. See Figure 9.8 for a spin dribble.

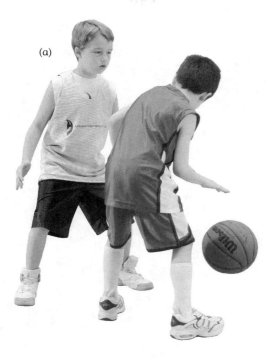

(a)

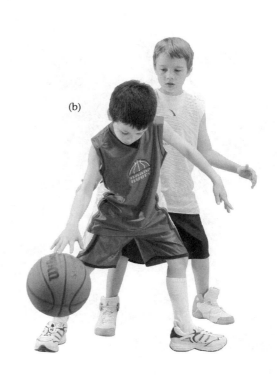

(b)

FIGURE 9.8

(a) To begin a spin dribble, the player quickly stops and reverse pivots. (b) He pulls the ball behind him as he spins. (c) He switches hands and explodes past the defender.

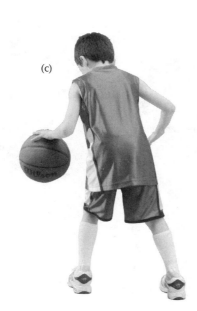

(c)

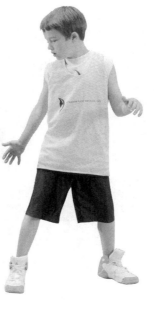

Half-spin Dribble

To execute a half-spin—to fake a defender into thinking the dribbler is going to execute a full spin dribble—the player begins executing a spin dribble as just described. Halfway through the dribble, instead of completing the spin, the dribbler returns to the original position and drives past his defender. See Figure 9.9 for a half-spin dribble.

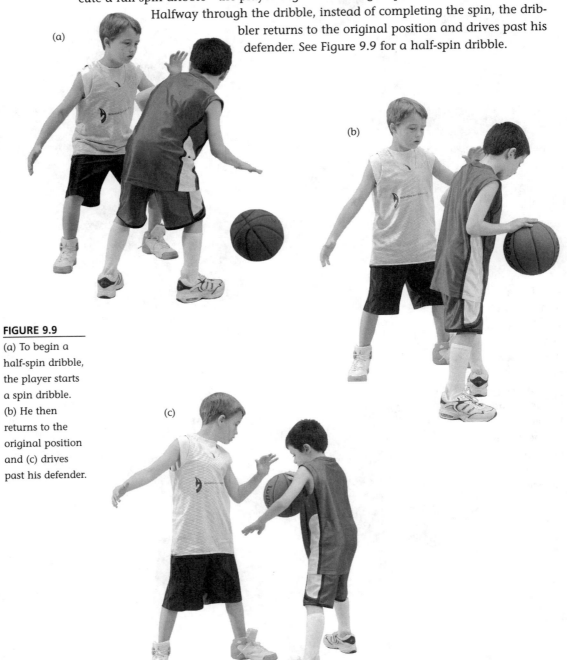

(a)

(b)

(c)

FIGURE 9.9

(a) To begin a half-spin dribble, the player starts a spin dribble. (b) He then returns to the original position and (c) drives past his defender.

Passing and Catching

Passing is another way to move the ball. It's a vital offensive weapon. A good passing team is difficult to defend because passes move faster than defenders. When you combine the ability to move to get open (by cutting and moving to open space) with good passing and able receiving, you'll create lots of opportunities to score.

There are four types of passes you should teach your players: the bounce pass, the chest pass, the overhead pass, and the baseball pass.

Bounce Pass

A *bounce pass* is useful in many situations, including when the receiver is on the move (which means his defender will be on the move, and thus have difficulty reaching down to deflect the pass), and when the defender is directly between the passer and the receiver.

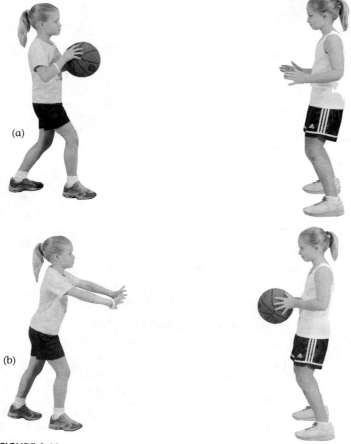

One way to pass the ball is to bounce it to a teammate. It's sometimes easier to bounce the ball past a defender than it is to pass the ball without bouncing it because it makes it harder for the defender to reach the ball.

To make a bounce pass, passers

1. Grasp the ball with both hands, using their fingers on the sides of the ball.

2. Take a step toward their target, if possible (see Figure 9.10a).

3. Push their arms forward, releasing the ball so it bounces about two-thirds of the way to their target, and so the ball bounces to about waist height of their teammate (see Figure 9.10b). The thumbs of the passer should be pointing in after releasing the ball.

(a)

(b)

FIGURE 9.10

(a) Stepping toward the target; (b) releasing the ball.

Sometimes the passer won't be able to step toward his target, but will have to pass around a defender (see Figure 9.11).

FIGURE 9.11

Making a bounce pass around a defender.

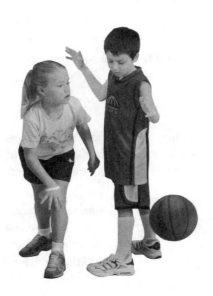
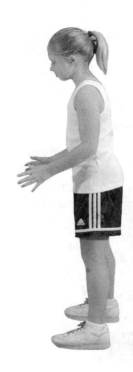

Chest Pass

A *chest pass* can be used when the passer has a clear path to the receiver. As with a bounce pass, the passer should

1. Grip the ball with her fingertips on the side of the ball.

2. Step toward her target (see Figure 9.12a).

3. Make a crisp pass to her teammate (see Figure 9.12b). As with the bounce pass, the passer's thumbs should be pointing in after releasing the ball.

note

The bounce pass should be about two-thirds of the way to the receiver because otherwise the pass will be too hard to handle (if it bounces too low) or too easy to steal (if it bounces too high). About two-thirds of the way to the target, with some decent zip on the ball, should get the job done.

The passer should snap the ball on a line from her chest area to the receiver's chest. Teach your players to quickly push straight out with their arms and snap their wrists as they release the ball. The pass shouldn't lazily loop toward the receiver because it will be too easy to steal. It also shouldn't come in so hard that the player can't catch it.

FIGURE 9.12

(a) Stepping toward the target; (b) making the chest pass.

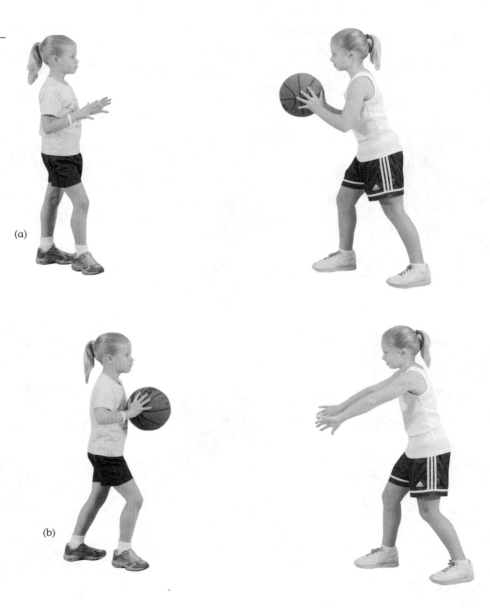

(a)

(b)

Overhead Pass

Players can use an overhead pass to pass the ball over a defender to a teammate. This type of pass is often used after securing a defensive rebound and passing the ball to a teammate to move the ball up the court.

To make an overhead pass, the player should

1. Hold the ball with two hands above his head (see Figure 9.13a).

2. Step toward his target (see Figure 9.13b).

3. Extend his arms and snaps his wrists as he releases the ball (see Figure 9.13c).

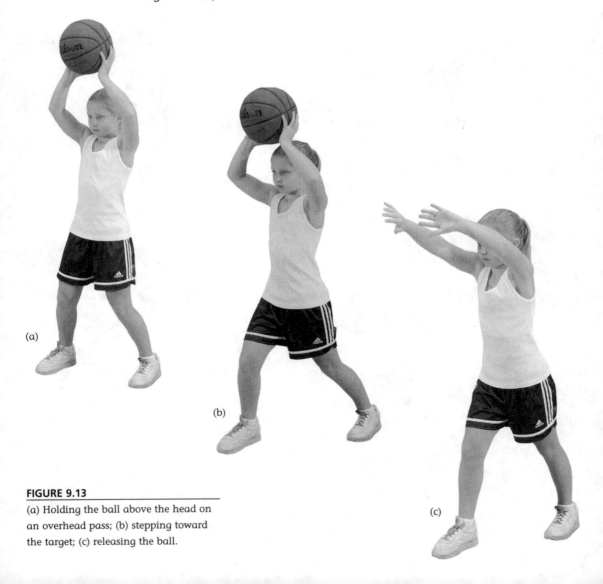

(a)

(b)

(c)

FIGURE 9.13

(a) Holding the ball above the head on an overhead pass; (b) stepping toward the target; (c) releasing the ball.

Baseball Pass

A *baseball pass* is a long pass, thrown baseball-style, usually covering at least half the court. This type of pass is used for a last-second out-of-bounds pass down the court and for some fast-break situations.

To make such a pass, the player brings the ball behind his head with one hand and throws the ball to his target with the same motion used for throwing a baseball. Players need to remember to lead their targets with this pass; if the target is moving, the player needs to throw to where the teammate will be when the ball arrives, not to where the teammate currently is.

tip

The baseball pass is difficult for younger players and for any player with small hands. It's hard to control because it is thrown with one hand, and it requires greater strength than other passes. Teach this pass only to players who possess the strength and control to use it. Most players under the age of nine will have difficulty throwing this pass.

Catching

Don't make the mistake of not teaching your players how to catch the ball. Inexperienced coaches think catching is a natural ability their players already have. Not so! Teach your players these techniques:

1. Give the passer a target by showing your hands in good catching position.
2. Come forward to meet the ball, especially if the ball might otherwise be knocked away by a defender.
3. Watch the ball all the way into your hands, using soft hands ("giving" with the ball) to cushion it.
4. Protect the ball from the defense as you catch it.
5. Make sure you catch the ball before you try to do something with it.

Shooting

You won't have to spend time motivating your kids to practice shooting! They'll be happy to spend ample amounts of time shooting because every player loves to score.

You *will* have to spend time teaching them the proper mechanics, though. And younger kids often have to *unlearn* improper mechanics they picked up in the backyard, hurling the ball at a too-high basket.

What types of shots should you teach? Let's focus on three: the outside shot, the layup, and the free throw.

Outside Shot

By *outside shot*, I mean shots taken from 12 to 15 feet or farther from the basket. Sometimes the shooter will use a jump shot for these shots (almost all older players will do so), and sometimes the shooter will keep her feet on the ground as she shoots (this is called a *set shot* because the player's feet are set).

Shooting involves the whole body and is done in one, continuous motion. The best shooters have a smooth, rhythmic form, starting with a dip of the knees, coming back up, and then extending the arms toward the basket and releasing the ball off the fingertips. The mechanics of shooting include these:

note

Most kids love three-pointers. But at younger ages, don't have them practicing lots of three-pointers as they attempt to hone their shooting technique. Shooting shots out of their range encourages poor form because they have to muscle the ball up to the hoop. Make sure they practice shots inside their range.

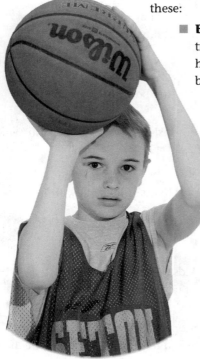

- **Ball**—Many times a player in a good scoring opportunity tries to shoot before he really has control of the ball because he's anxious to score. The first key is to have control of the ball. The fingers of the player's strong hand (the right hand for a right-hander) should be contacting the back side of the ball; the weak hand should be on the side, providing support and guidance (see Figure 9.14). The ball should be held about waist height prior to beginning the shot (see Figure 9.15a).

- **Legs**—To start the shooting action, the player dips his knees (see Figure 9.15b), and then pops them quickly back up. The power for shots comes through the leg action, not through the arms.

- **Arms**—As the legs straighten, the player brings the ball up with his elbow parallel to his body and pointing toward the basket (see Figure 9.15c). He extends his shooting arm and releases the ball by snapping his wrist toward the target (see Figure 9.15d).

FIGURE 9.14

Holding the ball in preparing to shoot.

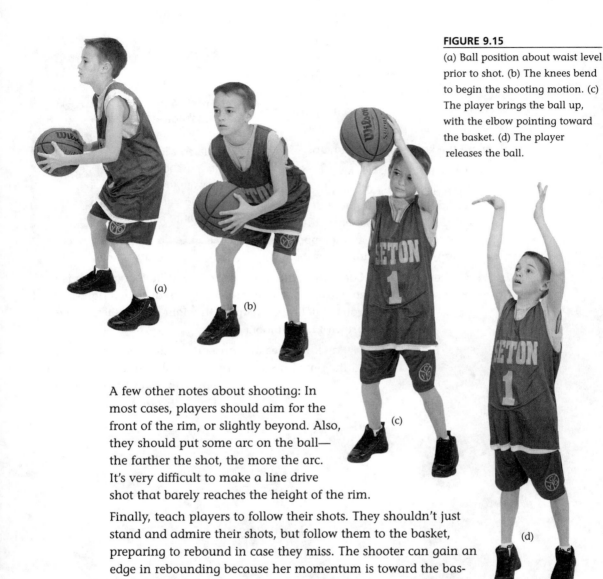

FIGURE 9.15

(a) Ball position about waist level prior to shot. (b) The knees bend to begin the shooting motion. (c) The player brings the ball up, with the elbow pointing toward the basket. (d) The player releases the ball.

A few other notes about shooting: In most cases, players should aim for the front of the rim, or slightly beyond. Also, they should put some arc on the ball—the farther the shot, the more the arc. It's very difficult to make a line drive shot that barely reaches the height of the rim.

Finally, teach players to follow their shots. They shouldn't just stand and admire their shots, but follow them to the basket, preparing to rebound in case they miss. The shooter can gain an edge in rebounding because her momentum is toward the basket, while her defender's is away from the basket, and because she knows where the shot is going. So if the shooter follows her shot, she can often get a rebound and be in position to make a follow-up shot.

Layup

Layups—short shots that are banked off the backboard—are common in youth basketball and are one of the most effective ways to score.

Layups often start with a dribble toward the basket, though not always. When the player with the ball sees an opening to the basket, he dribbles hard toward the hoop.

The ballhandler should dribble low and keep his front shoulder low as he drives to the basket. The rules allow the dribbler one step coming off the final dribble and then one more step without dribbling before the player has to release the ball.

Here are the keys to making layups:

- Drive to the basket. Most often, younger players will use their strong hands to dribble to the basket. As they gain skill and experience, they should also learn to drive to the opposite side, using their weak hand to dribble.

- Gather the ball in both hands and push off the opposite foot (see Figure 9.16a). After picking up the dribble and taking the final step, a right-handed shooter shooting a layup on the right side pushes off the court with his left foot.

- Raise the knee and arm on the shooting side (that is, the right knee and arm for a right-handed shooter) and jump up toward the hoop (see Figure 9.16b).

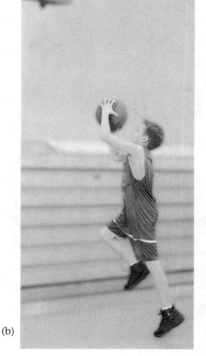

(b)

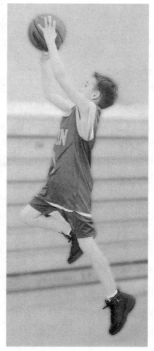

(b)

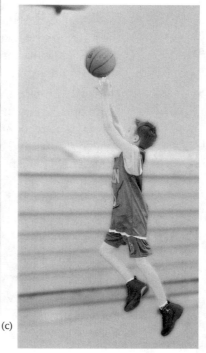

(c)

FIGURE 9.16

(a) Push off the opposite foot for a layup. (b) Raise the knee and arm on the shooting side. (c) Lay the ball softly off the backboard.

- Lay the ball softly on the backboard, with the palm turned inward and the fingertips pointing toward the basket, so the ball caroms into the basket (see Figure 9.16c). Players should take care not to use too much force in releasing the ball, as that will cause the ball to ricochet off the rim.

Free Throw

Players should develop a routine for their free throw shooting, approaching the free shots in the same way each time. This routine will help players focus on their task at hand and block out the things that might distract them. An example of a routine is to bounce the ball three times, getting a good feel for the ball, lining up the lines of the ball with the fingertips, taking a deep breath while focusing on the rim, and then bending the knees, coming up, and using the same shooting form as in shooting outside shots (except for keeping the feet on the floor).

Keys to shooting free throws include

- Pointing the front foot (the right foot for a right-handed shooter) toward the basket
- Squaring up the shoulders and hips to the basket
- Developing a routine that helps the player focus on the shot
- Using good shooting form, including bending the knees, coming up, extending the shooting arm, and releasing the ball with a snap of the wrist

tip

Teach your players to drive close to their defenders, not far from them (the dribbler has to be able to protect the ball from the defender, of course). The defender has to establish position and be stationary for the dribbler to be called for a charging foul. By driving close to the defender, this puts the defender in danger of committing a foul.

Rebounding

Rebounding is a critical skill to learn because it helps a team either gain or maintain control of the ball. It is both an offensive and defensive skill, but we'll cover rebounding mainly in this chapter, and just touch on a few highlights in the next chapter, which is on defense.

On offense, a rebound often means an immediate good scoring opportunity. On defense, a rebound means the opponents' scoring opportunity was snuffed out, and you now have a chance to move the ball down the court and score.

Shooting, passing, and dribbling call on fine motor skills that can take a long time to develop. Rebounding calls on gross motor skills that are more easily learned.

Rebounding is all about positioning, knowing how to use your body to block out and maintain position, having a sense for where the ball is going, hustling, and controlling the ball. Let's take a look at each key.

Initial Positioning

Generally the defensive player will have the initial advantage in gaining good position for a rebound because the defender is closer to the basket. The key here, of course, is to get in good rebounding position, which in most cases means the player is closer to the basket than her opponent.

For an offensive player to gain inside positioning, she must read her defender and use her quickness to get around her opponent. Sometimes a quick step in one direction and then a cut in the opposite direction can help the offensive player gain inside positioning.

A defender gains inside positioning by pivoting and facing the basket after a shot goes up.

Blocking Out

After positioning is gained, the most critical aspect of rebounding becomes blocking out (also called boxing out). When a player effectively blocks out her opponent, she uses her body as a screen to keep her opponent from getting around her.

Teach your players to make some contact with the player they're blocking out. Your players should spread their arms and legs wide and make contact with their rears to the opponents' bodies (see Figure 9.17). They should maintain contact with their opponents until releasing to go after the rebound.

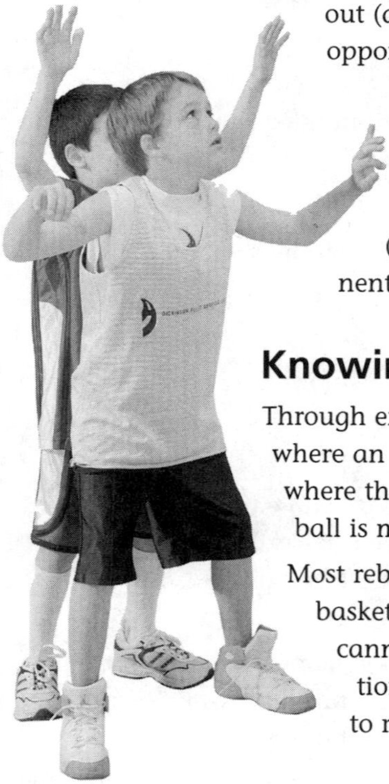

Knowing Where the Ball Is Going

Through experience, your players will begin to get a knack for knowing where an errant shot might go. They will be able to read the shot, seeing where the ball will strike the rim, and thus know approximately where the ball is most likely to go.

Most rebounds, when shot from outside, carom to the opposite side of the basket and at the same angle as the shot to the basket. If the player cannot get inside rebounding position, he should at least get a position beside his assignment and on the side where he expects the ball to ricochet.

FIGURE 9.17
Blocking out.

Hustling

Hustling is a big part of rebounding. Smaller players can use their bodies to block out and out-hustle bigger players, negating the size advantage of the bigger players. Much of rebounding is pure desire—who wants the ball more.

Controlling the Ball

Teach your players to aggressively jump for the ball after they have boxed out their opponent and see where the ball is going. A common mistake young players make is to watch the ball and wait for it to come to them. While they're waiting, their opponent might sneak in and secure the rebound.

So teach them to aggressively go after the ball (while making sure they control their bodies and don't foul an opponent; *over the back* is a common foul committed by overzealous rebounders who go over the back of their opponents in trying to grab a rebound). Players should use two hands in securing the ball, and bring the ball down to about chin level, with elbows out (see Figure 9.18).

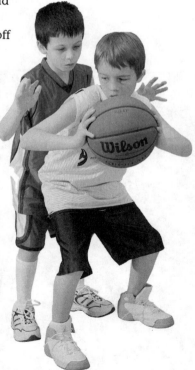

If a player secures an offensive rebound, she should look to first put the ball back up because she will most likely be close to the basket. If she can't get off a good shot (or draw a foul in trying a contested shot), she should look to pass to an open teammate.

If a player secures a defensive rebound, she should look to clear the ball to a teammate on the side, and not in the middle of the court, because the middle is more congested and a stolen pass could easily be converted into a layup or a short, open shot.

Passing Game

Sometimes younger players overlook the passing game. They get the ball and their immediate thought is either to shoot or dribble. The passing game can be an overlooked weapon. When teams rely primarily on dribbling to move the ball, they are doing the defense a favor because dribbling is much slower than passing.

Help your team to see the benefits of the passing game, and to understand some of its basics:

FIGURE 9.18

Securing the ball during a rebound.

■ **Pass and move to open spaces**—Many times a younger player will make a pass and then remain where she is, as if she has completed her duties for the time being. Instill in your players the need to move to open space, to find open teammates, and to maintain a court balance. But be careful how you describe court balance because if you say your players should be spread out over the court, they might each find an area and stay there. Instruct them to be moving, to find open space, and to always be ready to catch a pass as they're moving. And part of that movement should occur after passing.

■ **Deliver the right type of pass**—Sometimes a player who is *posted up*— near the basket with her back to the basket and a defender behind her—is open to receive a chest pass. But if the area is congested, a bounce pass or an overhead pass might work better. Knowing what type of pass to throw comes with experience. Guide your players in this area throughout the season.

■ **Pass away from the defender**—If a defender is on the right hip of a player, that player should receive a pass on her left side, rather than directly at her or to her right (see Figure 9.19). This allows her to use her body to shield the ball from the defender.

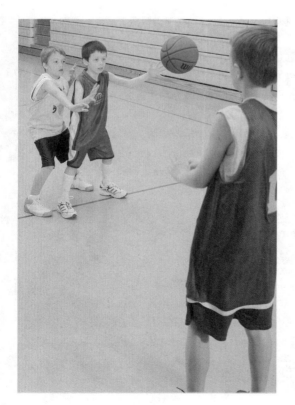

■ **Use some deception in passing**—Passes are often stolen because the defense can see well in advance where the pass is going. At this age I'm not advocating using lots of no-look or look-away passes, where the passer literally isn't looking at her target when she makes the pass, but I do recommend your players learn not to stare at their target for several seconds before passing. Part of this problem is alleviated with movement. When players are standing around and the passer stares at her receiver, that's an open invitation to a steal. When players are constantly moving and passers are looking to pass to teammates finding open space, the passing game improves.

FIGURE 9.19

Passing away from the defender.

Screens

Screens (also called picks) are a great strategy to use to get players open. A dribbler can use a screen to break free of her defender and be able to drive and shoot or pass off. A player without the ball can use a screen to get open, receive a pass, and get an open shot at the basket (see Figure 9.20).

FIGURE 9.20
Using a screen to break free for a shot.

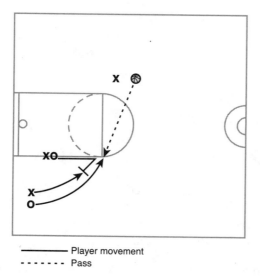

——— Player movement
- - - - - - Pass

To set a legal screen, a player has to be stationary. If the player makes contact with a defender while moving, the player setting the screen will be called for a foul. Here are the basics to setting a screen:

1. The screener gets into position to set a screen on a defender. The best position to set a screen is to the side and a little behind the defender, so the defender doesn't see the screen being set (see Figure 9.21).

2. The screener stands with legs spread about shoulder-width apart. Hands can be kept down or held at the chest.

3. The screener should brace himself for a collision because when it's set well, the defender doesn't see the screen, or catches it out of the corner of his eye at the last second.

4. The player moving past the screen should actually brush by his teammate. This leaves no space for the defender to slip through.

tip

Timing is important in screening. If the screen is set too early, the defender can see it and avoid it. If it's set too late, the screener risks being called for a foul for not being stationary. The ideal time to set a screen is just a second or two before it will be used.

The player receiving the screen should dip away from the screen before moving toward the screen. This timing needs to be coordinated. The screener can call out the name of the person being screened, or raise a fist or open hand near shoulder level to indicate when to move toward the screen.

FIGURE 9.21

The screen set here opens up the player coming off the screen for a pass.

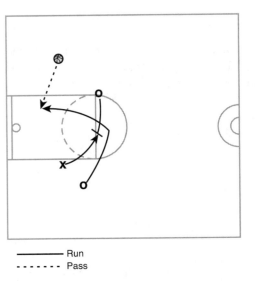

——————— Run
- - - - - - - Pass

5. After the screen is completed, the screener should look to roll toward the basket, or move toward open space, ready to receive a pass. (This pick-and-roll concept will be covered a little later in the chapter.) Often the screener will find himself open after setting a screen.

An important concept to teach your players is to screen away from the ball. The away portion means players look to set a screen on the side of the court opposite from where the ball is. For example, if the ball is on the left side of the court, players on the right side should look to set a screen. This allows a player to come off the screen and be moving toward the ball for a potential pass (see Figure 9.22).

FIGURE 9.22

Screening away from the ball.

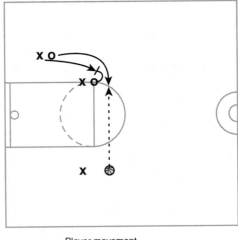

——————— Player movement
- - - - - - - Pass

Fast Break

Fast breaks are an exciting part of the game. The fast break involves most of the team and requires a variety of skills, including the abilities to dribble while running fast, to get down the court and fill open lanes, to make good passes while moving fast, and to convert while at or near top speed. To run the fast break effectively, it takes experienced and skilled players. Younger and less-experienced players can run the fast break, but expect them to make some mistakes as they learn how to put all the pieces together.

The fast break begins when the defense gains possession of the ball. The break can begin on a steal or on an inbounds play, but more often it begins on a defensive rebound. The rebounder makes an outlet pass to a teammate in the wing area, and that player either passes or dribbles the ball toward the middle of the court.

Generally the point guard brings the ball down the court because she is the best ball-handler. Her teammates are advancing down the court as well, filling the lanes on either side of the player with the ball.

Typically the player with the ball moves to the opponents' free throw line before deciding to pass off or to drive to the hoop. See Figure 9.23 for an example of a fast break.

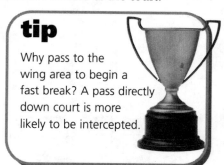

tip

Why pass to the wing area to begin a fast break? A pass directly down court is more likely to be intercepted.

FIGURE 9.23

The fast break.

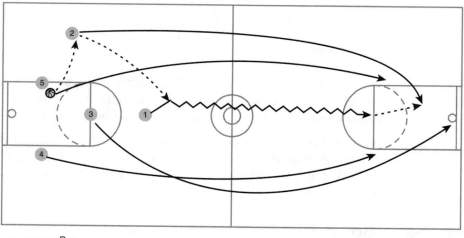

——————— Run
- - - - - - - Pass
WWWWWW Dribble

Basic Plays

Here we'll cover a few basic plays or concepts you can teach your players: the pick-and-roll, the give-and-go, and inbounds plays.

Pick-and-Roll

I alluded to the pick-and-roll a little bit ago. This is one of the oldest plays around, which is a testament to its effectiveness. It is also a relatively simple play. Player 1 sets a pick for Player 2; Player 1 then "rolls" to the basket, looking for a pass from Player 2 (see Figure 9.24).

FIGURE 9.24

Pick-and-roll.

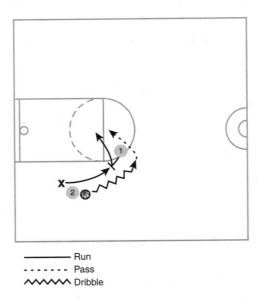

```
––––––––––  Run
- - - - - -  Pass
∿∿∿∿∿  Dribble
```

Why does this play work? Because the player who sets the pick is not the subject of the defense's attention. The focus is on picking up the player with the ball. The player who sets the pick is often left open as he cuts to the basket.

Teach your screeners to roll to the basket after setting a pick, and to be ready to receive a pass as they do. And teach your players who are using the pick to look for their teammate as they roll to the basket, and to be ready to pass if the player is open.

Give-and-Go

The give-and-go is also a play that has long been used in basketball. It is similar to the pick-and-roll in that a player executes it in a manner that puts the focus on a teammate, and then goes to the basket, looking for a pass.

In the give-and-go, Player 1 passes to Player 2, and then cuts to the basket, looking for a return pass. Depending on how tight the defense is, Player 1 can just cut straight to the basket (see Figure 9.25) or can use a fake step to get her defender off balance before cutting in a different direction to the basket (see Figure 9.26).

FIGURE 9.25
Cutting straight to the basket on a give-and-go.

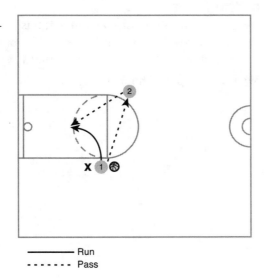

FIGURE 9.26
Using a fake on a give-and-go.

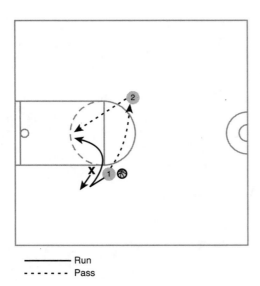

Inbounds Plays

Your team inbounds the ball numerous times during a game: after made baskets, after the ball goes out of bounds, and after turnovers and nonshooting fouls. Your players inbound the ball on their offensive end line, on their defensive end line, and on either sideline. Following are some plays to consider using in effectively getting the ball inbounds—and, in some cases, setting up immediate scoring opportunities.

At Your Own End of the Floor

When your team inbounds the ball on its offensive end line, it has a prime opportunity to score. Of course, the first concern is to get the ball safely inbounds, but if you can get a player open for a good shot off the inbounds pass, that's even better.

Figures 9.27 and 9.28 show inbounds plays that can result in an immediate basket.

FIGURE 9.27
An inbounds play under your own basket.

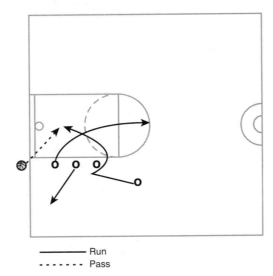

———— Run
------ Pass

FIGURE 9.28
Another inbounds play under your own basket.

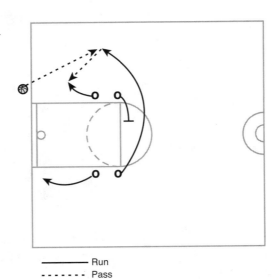

———— Run
------ Pass

At the Opponents' End of the Floor

If your league allows full-court presses and your opponent is pressing, it takes more work than normal to get the ball safely inbounds. Figure 9.29 shows one way to safely inbound the ball against a press.

On the Sideline

Figures 9.30 and 9.31 show a couple of options for inbounds plays along a sideline. Note that in Figure 9.30, Player 1 could go on either side of Player 2, who is setting a pick. In Figure 9.31, Player 1 is the primary option, Player 5 is a secondary option, and Players 3 and 4 are safety valves.

In general, you want a good passer to throw the ball inbounds, and you want to get it into the hands of a good ballhandler.

> **note**
>
> Remember, after a made basket, the player throwing the ball inbounds can run along the end line. On other inbounds plays, the player throwing the ball inbounds must keep a pivot foot on the floor.

FIGURE 9.29

Passing inbounds to beat a press.

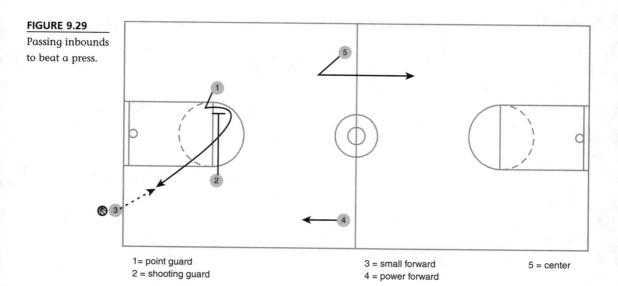

1 = point guard
2 = shooting guard

3 = small forward
4 = power forward

5 = center

An inbounds
play along the
sideline.

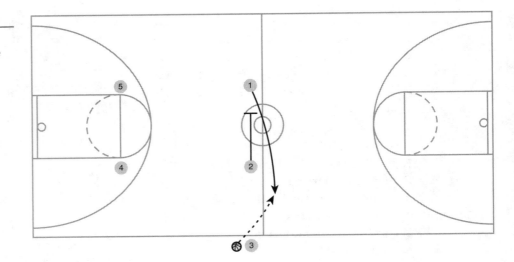

FIGURE 9.31
Another
inbounds play
along the
sideline.

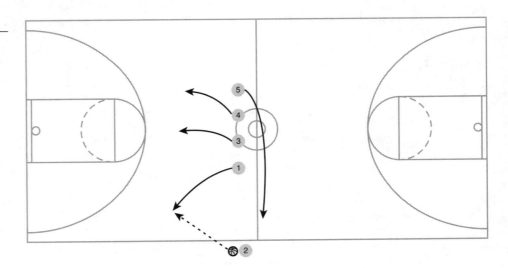

THE ABSOLUTE MINIMUM

This chapter covered the basic offensive skills of footwork, dribbling, passing, catching, shooting, and rebounding. It also covered tactical matters such as the passing game, setting screens, running the fast break, and other situations. Among the key points were

- Players should use a triple-threat stance from which they can shoot, pass, or dribble.

- Proper footwork, including pivots, cuts, jump stops, and jab steps, can create an advantage for players.

- Dribblers should use their fingertips, keep the ball low, protect it, and see the court as they dribble.

- Players should learn how to bounce pass, chest pass, overhead pass, and baseball pass, and know when to use each one.

- The mechanics of shooting involve a rhythm begun by bending the knees and popping them up. The elbow should be parallel to the body and pointing to the basket.

- Rebounding involves initial positioning, blocking out, knowing where the ball is going, and controlling it with two hands. Hustle and desire are important in rebounding.

- Players should set stationary screens to free a teammate either with or without the ball.

- To execute a fast break, the ball should be in the hands of a good ballhandler, with teammates filling the lanes on either side of the ballhandler.

- The pick-and-roll and give-and-go can create immediate scoring opportunities when executed properly.

IN THIS CHAPTER

- Defensive concepts
- Individual defensive skills
- Team defensive tactics

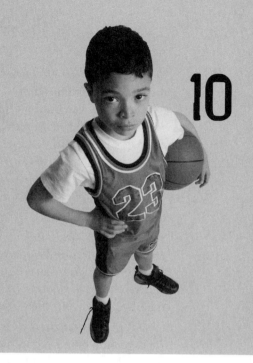

10

DEFENSIVE SKILLS AND TACTICS

Most players at the youth level (and often at higher levels as well) don't dream about being great defensive stars. They dream about raining in three-pointers, scoring lots of points, and being at the foul line for two shots with no time on the clock and down by one point.

Much of the glamour in basketball is focused on offense, but many games are won and lost on defense. An average-at-best team on offense can excel, and even win league titles, if they play topnotch defense.

Topnotch defense doesn't mean your players are blocking every shot in sight, or stealing the ball every time the opponents get their hands on it. It means your players know how to position themselves, how to cut off drives to the basket, how to defend against passes, how to get a hand up on shots, how to get through or around screens, and how to provide help when it's needed. It means they know not to reach in, not to go over the back on rebounds, not to go for head fakes. It means they know when to play tight and when to back off a bit. It means they know when to double-team and when to stick with their player. And it means they hustle and give full effort on defense, rather than mentally coasting and waiting until they get on offense again to be really tuned in to the game.

Yes, even great defenders commit fouls and make mistakes. You're not looking for perfection. You're looking for dedication and hustle, and the understanding for how to play solid defense.

You guessed it—that *understanding* part is your cue. Your players need to gain their defensive understanding from you. This chapter will help you teach them the defensive concepts, skills, and tactics they need to move toward becoming complete players. Maybe, after gaining an appreciation for the importance of defense, a few of them will even shift their dreams to game-winning blocked shots or steals.

Note that rebounding is as much a defensive skill as an offensive one, but because we covered rebounding in the previous chapter, we'll just quickly review a few basic rebounding concepts in this chapter.

Okay, on to the concepts, skills, and tactics of playing defense. Let's take a look at the concepts first.

Defensive Concepts

The concepts presented here are the underpinnings of playing solid, airtight defense. If your players get these concepts down, if they understand and consistently execute them to the best of their abilities, your team will quickly gain a reputation as a great defensive unit. It's much better to have players with only average skills who thoroughly understand the concepts, rather than players with superior ability who don't have a clue as to what they should be trying to do on defense.

Here, then, are seven concepts to instill in your players.

#1: Get Back Quick!

There's nothing more disheartening than to watch your team get beat on a fast break—especially if they get beat down the court simply from a lack of hustle.

When the other team gains possession of the ball, your players need to retreat quickly down to the other end of the floor. More precisely, they need to get down to the opposite end quicker than the opposition, and be ready to defend against a fast break or a quick attack.

Some players have a hard time making that quick transition from offense to defense. And good opponents will exploit that, and score lots of easy buckets. So, keep reinforcing a quick retreat until it is second nature with your players.

Here's an effective way to make this concept second nature: When you are scrimmaging on your half-court offense, have the defense fast break to the other end of the court when they rebound a missed shot. When the fast break is stopped (the fast break must get the shot, not the secondary break or the set offense), the original offense again operates from the other end of the floor. Continue this in a controlled scrimmage atmosphere.

note

Much of a player's ability to shine on defense relies on his concentration, attitude, intensity, and physical conditioning. Kids who don't have a great shot or superior ball-handling abilities can excel on defense and contribute significantly to the team effort.

#2: Apply Pressure

Teach your players to play active, aggressive defense. The more pressure they can apply to the ballhandler, without fouling, the better. Without that pressure, the ballhandler is comfortable and in charge, and can be on the attack. With constant pressure, much of the ballhandler's focus is spent on maintaining possession. She will have a harder time penetrating the lane and dishing off, or seeing open teammates.

Three keys to applying pressure are to maintain good positioning, to use a slide step, and to get a hand up on all shots. You'll learn more about these in "Individual Defensive Skills" later in the chapter.

#3: Cut off Passing Lanes

If your team can't cut off passing lanes, the opponents can quickly move the ball into scoring position. Your players have to recognize what passing lanes are, and know how to close them down.

Teach your players to use peripheral vision when they're guarding a player without the ball. Defenders away from the ball should know where the ball is, and stay between the player they're guarding and the basket. They should get a hand and a foot in the passing lane (see Figure 10.1). When *ball side*—that is, when on the side of the court that the ball is on—the defender should be just a step or two away from his assignment, facing the ball with hand, leg, and head in the passing lane. When *weak side,* the defender stays low, points to the ball with one hand and to his assignment with the other, and uses peripheral vision to see both the ball and his assignment.

note

What do ball side and weak side mean? Envision a court with a line drawn down the center of it, from under one basket to under the basket at the other end. *Ball side* is the side of the court that the ball is on; *weak side,* which is also referred to as *help side,* is the other side of the court.

FIGURE 10.1

The defender gets a hand and a foot in the passing lane.

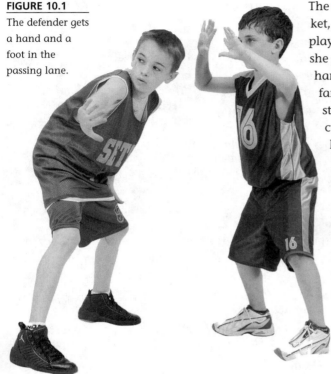

The closer the defender's player is to the basket, the closer she should defend. If her player is within 12 feet or so of the basket, she should be within a couple of feet, with a hand in the passing lane. If her player is farther away, she can sag off a little, but still be ready to move with her player and cut off any passes or movement that puts her opponent in good position to receive a pass and score.

How much should they sag off? On the weak side, the defender should be one step off the line between his assignment and the ball, and two-thirds of the distance from the ball (see Figure 10.2). On the ball side, your defenders should be in the passing lane as described in "Cut off Passing Lanes."

FIGURE 10.2

The defender gets one step off the line between his assignment and the ball, and two-thirds of the distance from the ball.

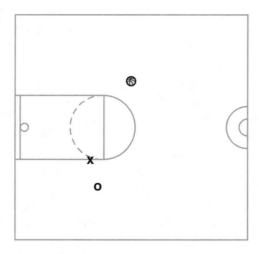

Sagging off on the weak side, one step off the line between assignment and ball, and two-thirds of the distance from the ball. As your players gain experience, they'll more readily recognize passing lanes and be ready to defend against them. This doesn't mean they won't allow passes to be received; it means they will begin to minimize the number of passes that penetrate their defense and leads to advantages for the offense.

#4: Deny the Ball Down Low

One of the most critical areas to defend is down low, near the basket. If your team allows the ball to get down low, the chance for a basket (and perhaps a foul on your team, as well) rises.

Players guarding opponents in the post or lane should play tight defense, essentially right on top of the player they're guarding, without fouling. Defenders in the lane can't afford to sag off their player, unless it's to move over to help guard another opponent who has the ball and is driving to the hoop or is about to shoot.

Otherwise, defenders down low should stick tight to their opponent. When the offensive player is ball side and within six feet of the basket, the defender can *front* the player—literally stand in front of him, a hand up to prevent a pass going over the top (see Figure 10.3). Fronting a player usually isn't a good idea if the player is farther out because the passer can lob a pass over the top of the defender.

#5: Don't Commit Unnecessary Fouls

Not committing unnecessary fouls begs the question, "Are there *necessary* fouls to commit?" If not necessary, you could at least call some fouls appropriate. For example, if a player is going to get an easy layup, rather than just give the opponents the two points, you could foul the player and make her "earn" the points at the free throw line. Or a good defender who often is successful at stealing the ball might foul while attempting a steal; this is part of the risk involved. Or you might commit a foul toward the end of the game to stop the clock and get the ball back if you're losing.

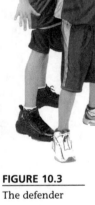

FIGURE 10.3
The defender fronts the opponent.

Unnecessary fouls, on the other hand, are the type that neither benefits your team nor have reason to be committed. These fouls include reaching in, going over the back, holding, pushing, setting a moving screen, and hand checking, to name a few.

Realize, of course, that fouling is a part of the game, and you can't ask your players to play tight, aggressive defense without expecting

warning

If you instruct your players to foul an opponent instead of allowing an easy layup, make sure you are very clear that the foul should not be overly hard or severe; you don't want to injure the other player. You just want to stop the shot. This strategy is probably best employed by players 10 and older.

them to commit fouls. The point here is to try to minimize the fouls players have some control over. For example, players should

- Work for positioning, or move around their opponent, rather than just going "over the back" and making contact with him.

- Pick the right time to steal. Reaching in is almost always a bad thing to do because it usually looks like a foul, even if the defender makes no contact. Instead, defenders should focus on intercepting passes and making steals when the dribbler isn't shielding the ball with her body.

- Get in position and use their bodies to check the progress of an offensive player, rather than holding or pushing.

#6: Provide Help

There will be plenty of opportunities for your players to help each other on defense: An opponent slips by her defender and is driving to the hoop (see Figure 10.4). A defender gets out of position and his opponent receives a pass and is open for a shot (see Figure 10.5). A taller and stronger opponent receives a pass down low, and has been easily scoring in such situations when one-on-one with the player who is defending her (see Figure 10.6).

FIGURE 10.4

Defender X2 provides help on a drive.

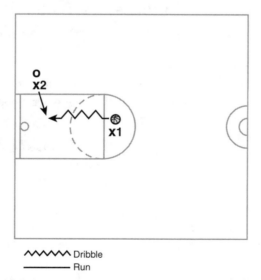

These are just a few of the situations that call for defenders to help each other. For players to provide good help on defense, they need to be aware not only of the player they're guarding, but of the action as it unfolds around them. They need to sense when a teammate might need help, and to be alert at all times to provide it.

They need to know when to provide it. They should always provide it if the opponent is likely to score if they don't provide the help. They shouldn't provide it if in doing so it doesn't diminish the advantage for the opposition. For example, if a defender moves over to double-team a player and in doing so leaves his own player wide open for a pass near the basket, that's not a wise decision.

And they need to communicate. Defenders shouldn't just hope their teammates see they need help; they should shout, "Help!" That leads us to our final defensive concept.

FIGURE 10.5
Defender X2 provides help when a defender is out of position.

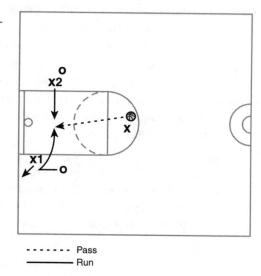

- - - - - - - Pass
————— Run

FIGURE 10.6
Defender X2 provides help on a player down low.

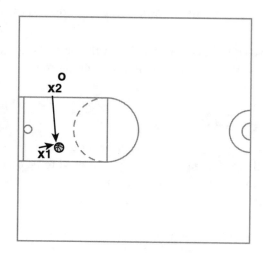

#7: Communicate!

Your help on defense isn't going to be too strong if your players don't communicate with each other. Players need to talk to alert each other as to where the ball is and what's going on. Practice good communication because it's a vital aspect of team defense, and it doesn't come naturally for many kids.

Here are a few examples of when and how players should communicate:

- When a screen is being set, the player about to be screened usually doesn't see the screen. A teammate—generally the one who is guarding the offensive player setting the screen—should shout "Screen left!" or "Screen right!" The "left" or "right" is from the perspective of the defender being screened. "Screen left" means he should watch for a screen being set to his left side.

- Another option in communicating on screens is for the defender who sees the screen coming to shout "Switch!" This means the two defenders involved in the play—the defender being screened and the defender guarding the player who is setting the screen—swap defensive assignments. (You'll learn more about the various options in "Defend Against Screens" later in the chapter.)

- In getting back to defend against a fast break, often there are a couple of defenders against two or three offensive players. The defenders should shout out, by the player's number, which player they will take: "I've got 17!" (When it's a 3-on-2 situation, the two defenders play the two offensive players who pose the greatest threat.)

- If a defender is beaten on a drive to the basket, or anywhere else that poses a threat to the defense, she should call out "Help!" One of her teammates should shift over to pick up her player, and other teammates adjust accordingly.

- As the ball is received by an offensive player, the defender guarding the new ballhandler can shout out "Ball!" to alert teammates to the ball's location.

Individual Defensive Skills

So far we've talked about a number of concepts that should guide your players' defensive efforts. To aid them in their efforts, they also need to be able to execute specific skills. In this section we'll look at a number of defensive skills you'll want to help your players develop.

Maintain Good Positioning

Stealing the ball, blocking a shot, taking a charge, rebounding, and stopping a drive call on a variety of skills and attributes—quick hands and feet, good jumping ability, and size and strength, not to mention the intestinal fortitude it requires to take a charge.

They also have a common denominator: The defender was in good position to make the play.

The fundamental set of skills in playing good defense revolves around positioning. If a defender can't maintain good positioning, he's going to be a defensive liability, no matter how athletic he might be.

There are several keys to defensive positioning, depending on the situation. We'll consider these issues:

- Defense on the ball
- Defense off the ball on a ball-side player
- Defense off the ball on a weak-side player

Defense on the Ball

Teach your defenders to stay low, bent at the knees and waist, about a step away from the player with the ball (see Figure 10.7). The defender's hands should be out from her body, from waist to chest height, ready to reach out to tip a pass. As mentioned earlier, the defender should have a hand and a foot in the passing lane. The feet should be a little wider apart than shoulder width, with the player's weight up on her toes and not flat-footed, so she is ready to move in any direction.

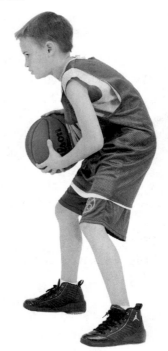

The defender should focus on the ballhandler's midsection so he isn't faked out, and stay between the player and the basket. The primary goal is to not allow the player to dribble where he wants to or to have an open lane for passing to a teammate. The defender should try to beat the dribbler to the spot where he is dribbling, thus cutting off a drive to the basket and forcing him to pick up his dribble or move to a less-threatening area. After the

FIGURE 10.7

The defender stays low, hands out, in on-the-ball defense.

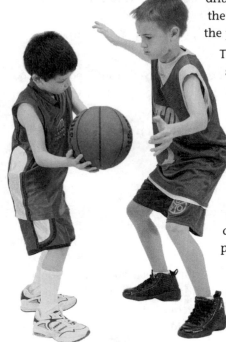

dribbler has picked up his dribble, the defender should crowd the player and make it difficult to pass by getting a hand in the passing lane (see Figure 10.8).

The defender on the ball should keep his hands on the same plane as the ball, moving his hands as the attacker moves the ball up and down and around. This will help the defender to get his hands on a pass or shot.

Defense off the Ball on a Ball-Side Player

When guarding a player who is on ball side and who does not have the ball, the defender should look to deny the pass as described in "Cut off Passing Lanes." The defender should be just a step or two away from his assignment, facing the ball with hand, leg, and head in the passing lane.

When playing off the ball, your defenders should maintain awareness of not only their player, but where the ball is and how the play is developing around them. They should know where the ball is and be ready to provide help if needed.

FIGURE 10.8
The defender crowds the player after he has picked up his dribble, making it difficult to pass.

Defense off the Ball on a Weak-Side Player

When guarding a player who is weak side and does not have the ball, the defender stays low, points to the ball with one hand and to his assignment with the other, and uses peripheral vision to see both the ball and his assignment. This position was shown in Figure 10.2 in "Cut off Passing Lanes."

Use a Slide Step

A defender uses a *slide step* to maintain good positioning whether the opponent goes to the left or right. In sliding to the right, the player moves her right foot first, and then her left foot slides over, *never crossing the right foot*. As she moves, she maintains her stance, keeping low, ready to change direction at any time. If players cross their feet as they slide, they risk getting their feet tangled up, especially if they have to quickly change direction.

tip

A common reason defenders get beat by a player with the ball is because they watch the ball or the player's head or feet. Train your youngsters to watch the player's midsection. The midsection doesn't lie, and the midsection moves the least during fakes. They should focus on the belly because whatever direction the midsection is going, that's where the player is going.

Get Hands up on Shots

It's much more difficult for players to shoot if they have a hand near their face. Remind your players that when they jump and get a hand up to contest a shot, they need to make sure they don't make contact with the shooter (see Figure 10.9). They can, of course, make contact with the *ball*. But aggressively challenging the shot without fouling will make it harder for the shooter, even if there's no chance the defender can block the shot.

Go for the Steal

One of the most exciting plays on defense is a steal—especially if it leads to a break-away bucket at the other end. A steal can lift your team's spirits, swing the momentum their way, and get some quick points on the board.

tip

After players get the hang of playing good defense and maintaining good positioning, they can use their bodies to force ballhandlers to go one way or the other. For example, a defender can overplay one side to force a player to dribble toward the sideline. Defenders can also use this strategy to force dribblers to use their weak hand. For example, a defender can overplay a right-handed dribbler to the right side to try to force her to go left and use her left hand.

The key is to know *when* to attempt a steal and how to go about it. First, when *not* to attempt a steal: You want your players to put pressure on the dribbler, but not to reach in (to reach around the body of the dribbler to try to swipe the ball away): Even if they don't touch the dribbler, it almost always *looks* like they do, and a referee generally will call a foul. Certainly a defender should try to steal the ball if the dribbler is not protecting the ball with his body, but as players progress, this type of opportunity will be fairly rare.

Steals are more often made off passes than off dribbles. And the opportunities will be there if players look for them. Just as in rebounding, desire and attitude have a lot to do with a player's ability to steal. Your players have to *want* the ball, be *looking* for it, and *react* to it at just the right time. Quickness and proper positioning are also key attributes.

Many steals are a bit of a cat-and-mouse game, wherein the defender lies in waiting, appearing not to be a threat, and then

FIGURE 10.9

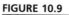

The defender gets a hand up to contest a shot.

times his strike at just the right moment, anticipating the pass to the player he's guarding (see Figure 10.10).

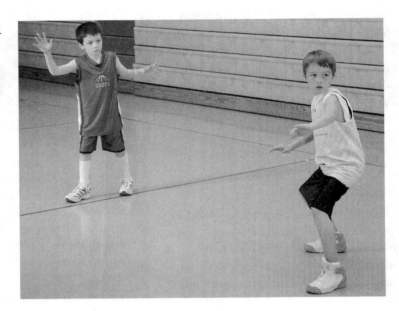

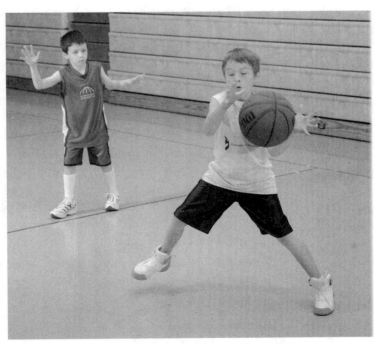

Box Out to Rebound

We covered rebounding in the previous chapter, but boxing out (or blocking out) is a key element to it, and one that you need to drill home with your players.

Defensive players have the inside edge on rebounding because they're closer to the basket. After a shot goes up, the defender pivots and boxes out her opponent, spreading her arms and legs wide and making contact with her rear against her opponent's body. She should maintain contact with her opponent until she releases to go after the rebound.

Team Defensive Tactics

Team tactics involve the ways teammates work together to defend. In this section we'll look at how to defend against screens, when and how to double-team the player with the ball, how to employ a full-court press, and a few basics on playing a player-to-player defense and a zone defense.

Defend Against Screens

Defenders have two basic options in defending against screens on the ball: They can stay with their players, meaning the defender being screened must "fight through" the screen or go around it, or the two defenders involved can switch players.

The ideal is to stay with their players. No one gets confused about who's guarding whom, and there aren't any last-second changes that can result in an advantage for the offense while the defense adjusts.

To fight through a screen, the defender steps between the screener and his player and moves through without fouling (see Figure 10.11).

FIGURE 10.11

The defender steps between the screener and his player and stays with his player.

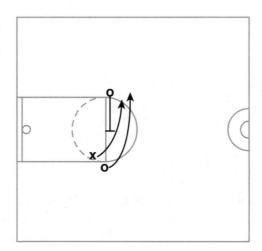

A defender should go around a screen when he sees he can't fight through it without fouling. In this case, he steps behind the screener and stays with his player (see Figure 10.12).

FIGURE 10.12

The defender steps behind the screen and stays with his player.

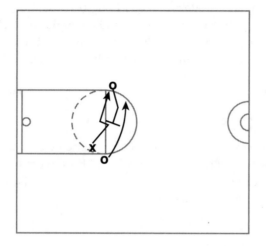

However, there are times when a screen is set up so effectively that it might be better to switch, so long as the switch is clearly and loudly communicated in time (see Figure 10.13). The defender originally covering the player setting the screen calls out "Switch!" if he believes his teammate can't get through or go around the screen to cover the other player, especially if the other player is the ballhandler.

FIGURE 10.13

The defender on the screener calls out "Switch!" The defenders switch and pick up their new assignments.

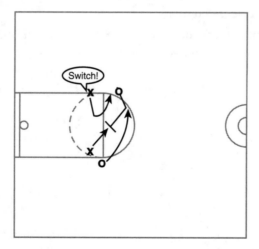

Teach your players to watch for the screener to roll toward the basket after setting the pick. Also, for older players, teach the defender who is guarding the screener to momentarily pop out to slow down the dribbler, while still keeping an eye on the screener, as his teammate fights through or goes around the screen and picks up his opponent again (see Figures 10.14).

FIGURE 10.14

The defender on the screener pops out to slow down the dribbler. The two defenders continue guarding their original players.

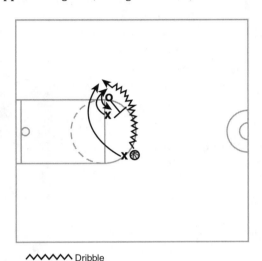

∿∿∿∿ Dribble

Defending against screens takes experience, practice, and timely communication to know which way to go. Screens are great to work on in practice because they give both the offense and the defense a chance to learn how to execute. Encourage your defenders to stay with their players when possible and to recognize when it's better to switch.

Double-team When Appropriate

Your players should watch for opportune moments to double-team the ballhandler. There are many times in which double-teaming can be especially effective. One example is to help stop a skilled offensive player, particularly when that player has the ball near the basket. The goal here is to stop a basket. You might say to your players in the huddle, "If number 24 gets the ball in the post, I want the nearest defender to help Kari out, even if Kari is in good position."

Another example when double-teaming is appropriate is to put pressure on a dribbler who has picked up her dribble, particularly when she is near any boundary line: a sideline, the end line, or the half-court line. The goal here is to directly steal the ball or make the player throw a pass that can be intercepted.

With this type of double-teaming, defenders need to have a sense for the right moment and quickly respond; otherwise the offensive player will have passed the ball and the opportunity will be gone. The right moment is when the player has picked up her dribble, when she's near one or more boundary lines, and when a secondary defender is near enough that she can quickly come over and apply pressure along with the defender who is already guarding the player with the ball.

Defenders should try to seal off any possible pass without reaching in and fouling (see Figure 10.15).

This play is most effective when employed against a ballhandler who is not a good passer, but it can work against even the best ballhandlers. The key is for your players to recognize when that pressure can be applied, when it can be most effective, and to seize the opportunity when it arises.

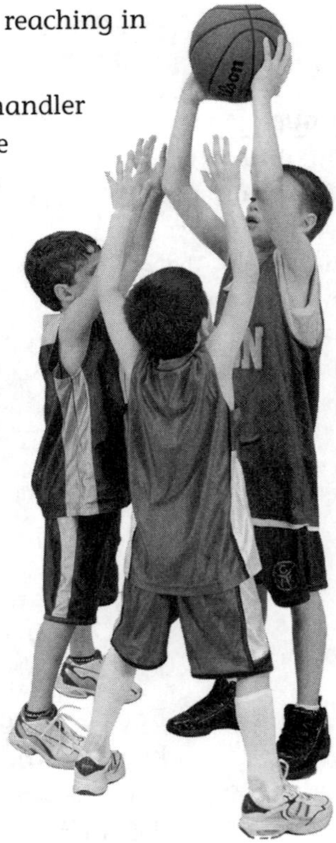

Use a Full-court Press

If you're coaching younger players, it's likely your league doesn't allow full-court pressing. But if you're coaching older players (11- and 12-year-olds), this is an option you might consider in applying pressure to create turnovers.

In a full-court press you put continuous pressure on the ball. Usually this begins with pressuring the inbounds passer. The opposing guards are of primary importance, as they are the ones most often called upon to bring the ball up the court. There are a variety of presses, most of which employ a trapping element in which the defenders look to double-team the ballhandler.

Usually one or two defenders stay back to guard against an easy basket, should the offense break the press. These defenders should also be alert for long passes over the press; such passes can often be intercepted.

FIGURE 10.15
Defenders double-team and make it difficult to pass.

To run an effective full-court press, you need players who are experienced, quick, and who work together well as a team. Otherwise, a press could backfire and could result in easy baskets for the opposition.

Use a Player-to-Player Defense

Most youth teams use a player-to-player defense, in which each player is matched against one opponent—guards versus guards, forwards versus forwards, and center versus center. This defense is more fun to play, and less confusing than a zone. In a zone, defenders often are unsure of what to do when the ball is away from their zone, and they tend to be inactive. In player-to-player, the defenders know at all times that they are to be guarding their assigned opponent, staying between him and the basket, denying the ball or defending against the ballhandler if their player receives a pass.

Use a Zone Defense

I recommend you use a zone defense sparingly, if at all, at the youth level. Perhaps occasionally you might consider using a zone. A zone is effective in guarding against

■ Quick guards that can easily penetrate and drive to the hoop

■ A dominant inside force

■ A team that has the upper hand in individual match-ups

Figure 10.16 shows four types of zones. If the opponents have good outside shooters and you want to play a zone, playing a 2-3 or a 2-1-2 would be better because you would have two defenders out front to stop outside shots. If you're more concerned about the opponents' forwards and center, pack the defense in a 1-3-1 or a 1-2-2. These provide more coverage in the lane.

FIGURE 10.16
(a) 2-1-2 zone.
(b) 1-3-1 zone.
(c) 2-3 zone.
(d) 1-2-2 zone.

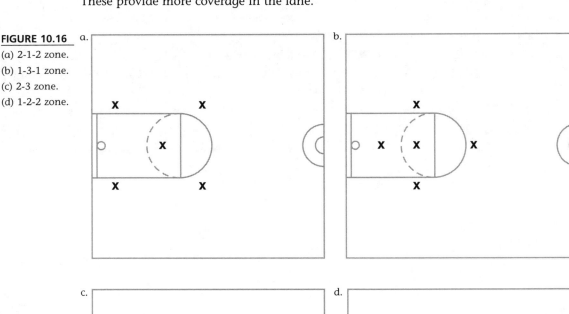

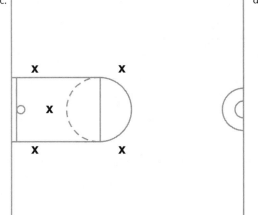

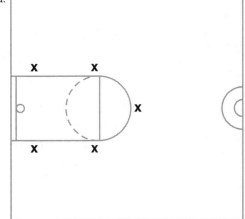

THE ABSOLUTE MINIMUM

This chapter focused on the skills and tactical understanding your players need to develop to play good defense. Among the key points were

■ Your players must learn defensive concepts, including getting back quickly in transition, applying pressure to the ball, cutting off passing lanes, and denying the ball down low.

■ In addition, they need to learn to not commit unnecessary fouls, to provide help when needed, and to communicate well with their teammates.

■ They need to work on individual skills, including maintaining good on-the-ball and off-the-ball defense, using slide steps to move laterally, and getting hands up on shots.

■ They also need to learn how to effectively block out to rebound and know when and how to go for a steal.

■ Team tactics they need to learn include defending against screens, double-teaming when appropriate, and using a full-court press, if rules allow and if you have the personnel to do so.

■ Finally, they need to learn how to work together as a unit in both player-to-player defenses and, on occasion, in zone defenses.

11

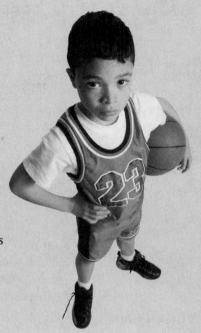

Games and Drills

Now we get to what many coaches love—games and drills to use to help their players improve their abilities to execute the skills and tactics of basketball.

Use these 23 games as they are, adapt them to fit your needs, or use them to spur you on to creating your own games and drills. Know, too, that you can find many games elsewhere, including online. There is no lack of games out there. The challenge is to use games and drills that will benefit your players the most. Many games are boring, make kids stand in line for a long time, or aren't very effective in helping kids practice skills they will use in real contests. Steer clear of those types of games.

Instead, use games that put your players in game-like situations, that are fun, that call on them to execute the skills and tactics they will need to perform in real games, and that keep them active and not standing around waiting a long time for their turn.

Good luck in your season. Enjoy it, and help your players enjoy the great sport of basketball!

Dribbling Games

Here are three games to help your players improve their dribbling skills. Remember to focus on good form and to provide helpful tips as they practice.

Game One

Name	On the Move
Purpose	To execute two basic dribbling moves and counters to defensive moves
Setup	Have your players line up in two lines near mid-court, one line facing each basket (see Figure 11.1). You stand near the top of the key at one basket, with your assistant at the top of the key at the other basket. It's best if each player has a ball, but you can run the drill with only two basketballs.
Description	The first player in each line begins dribbling toward the coach. The player executes the crossover dribble as he gets near the coach. Overplay the dribbler to help him learn when to execute the crossover.
	After dribbling past the coach, the player goes to the back of the other line. The next two times through the drill he executes

- The spin
- The counter to the spin—the half spin

FIGURE 11.1

Setup and execution for On the Move.

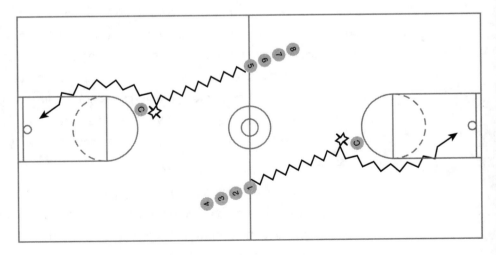

Notes	■ To make the drill more difficult, require players to use their "off" hand to dribble and execute the moves.

- Overplay the two basic moves, and fake overplaying one side before jumping into an overplay on the opposite side so the players can execute the counter moves. This teaches the "when" of executing those moves.

- Younger players might only be able to learn the crossover and the spin.

Game Two

Name	Dribble Tag
Purpose	For players to control their dribble while being harassed
Setup	Divide your players into equal numbers, half on one side of the court, half on the other side. Call one set of players Xs and the other Os. Every player has a ball (see Figure 11.2).
Description	The Xs are "it" and try to tag the Os by deflecting their ball away from them while all the players are dribbling. All dribblers must stay within the three-point arc. If the ball is deflected beyond the arc, they are "tagged." After the Xs have deflected all the balls out of their respective arcs, the Xs and Os exchange duties.

FIGURE 11.2
Setup for
Dribble Tag.

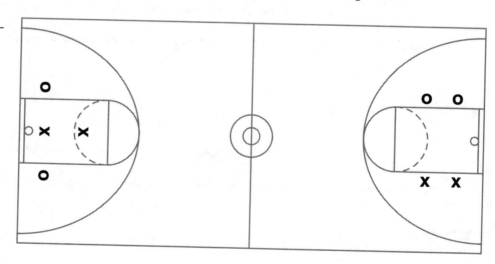

Notes	- You can do this as a one-on-one drill, where each individual game ends when a dribbler is tagged, or you can have the dribblers remain in the game after being tagged and become another "it," meaning that at the end all but one dribbler would be "it."
	- To make the game more fun, have a contest to see which team deflects the other team's balls out of the arc the quickest.

- To make the game more difficult, have the Xs dribble with their off hand while the Os dribble with their favored hand.

- To make the game even more difficult, have the Xs dribble with their favored hand while the Os dribble two balls at once.

Game Three

Name	Dribbling Relay
Purpose	To teach players to handle the ball with both hands and to refine their speed dribble
Setup	Line up players in two equal lines at one end of the court (see Figure 11.3). The front player in each line has a ball.
Description	The first player in each line begins a speed dribble down the floor. When the players reach the far end line, they spin dribble and then resume speed dribbling down the floor to the starting end line. The dribblers then pass to the next player in line, and go to the end of their respective lines.

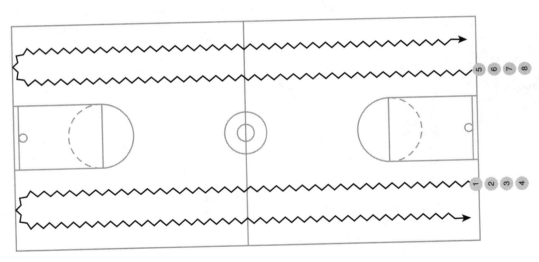

FIGURE 11.3

Setup and execution for Dribbling Relay.

Notes	■ To make the relay more fun, see which team finishes first with all players dribbling down and back.
	■ To make it more difficult, have the players dribble to the far end line, do a jump stop, pivot, and then dribble back to the starting free throw line, jump stop, and chest pass (or bounce pass) to the next player in line.

Passing Games

Here are a couple of games to sharpen your team's passing skills. They also help to work on defending against passes.

Game One

Name	Monkey in the Middle
Purpose	To practice various types of passes
Setup	Divide the team into squads of 3 players each. Place these squads about 15 feet apart anywhere on the court (see Figure 11.4).
Description	This is a two-part drill. You can do only Part A, only Part B, or both parts.

- In Part A, the three players pass the ball clockwise or counterclockwise, executing whatever type of pass you call out.

- In Part B, one of the three players is a defender. The defender keeps her arms in motion and her hands in the plane of the ball. Passers will often have to fake a pass or get the ball deflected. The players rotate so each can play defense.

FIGURE 11.4

Setup for Monkey in the Middle.

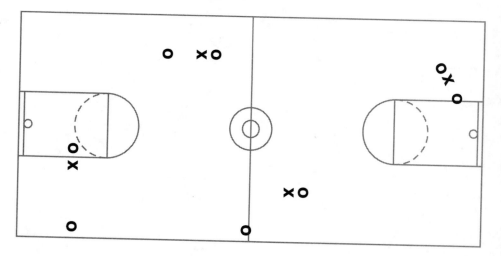

Notes

- To make Part B more fun, keep count of the number of deflections by each player during a timed period (two minutes is good). Have two players execute passes for two minutes and then rotate.

- This game is also effective in teaching defenders to keep a hand in the passing lane.

Game Two

Name	Keep It Moving
Purpose	To practice basic passes
Setup	Divide the squad into two groups, one on each end of the floor (see Figure 11.5). Designate three offensive players and two defenders in each group. Station one of the offensive players at the free throw line and the other two about three feet outside each of the two blocks near the basket. One defender is on the ball and the other is between the two receivers.
Description	This is a two-part drill. You can do Part A before moving into Part B, or just do Part B by itself.

- In Part A, use only three passers (rotate the other two players in after several passes). They pass the ball between each other, using the type of pass you call out.

- In Part B, one of the defenders is on the ball, arms in motion, hands in the plane of the ball; the other defender is between the two receivers attempting to steal or deflect any errant or poorly-thrown pass. After several passes, rotate the two defenders to offense and two of the offensive players to defense.

FIGURE 11.5

Setup for Keep It Moving.

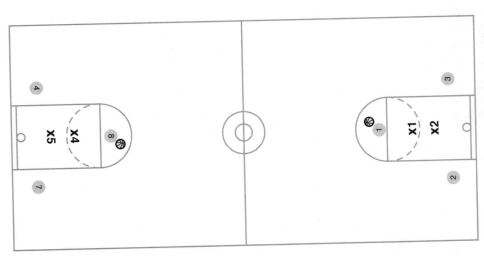

Notes	

- You can make a game out of this by giving a time limit and counting the number of deflections. The offensive team with the least number of deflections is the winner. (To focus on the defense, the defensive team with the most deflections wins.) Or you could require a certain number of deflections (three is a good number) before switching from offense to defense.

■ This game also helps defenders learn to play zone and to shoot the gaps for steals.

Shooting Games

Here are two games to help your players sharpen their shooting skills.

Game One

Name	Shooting Angle
Purpose	To practice correct shooting form
Setup	Divide the squad into two equal groups, half on one end of the court, half on the other end. Give each player a ball. Set the players up in each of five shooting angles: from the baseline left, from the baseline right, from the 45° angle left, from the 45° angle right, and from straight in front of the basket. See Figure 11.6 for the shooting angles.
Description	Each player begins at a different angle and begins shooting in the "A" position. After making the basket, the player steps back one step and shoots from the "B" position at the same angle. The player continues until he makes all four shots at that angle, and then he moves to a different angle.

FIGURE 11.6

Shooting angles for Shooting Angle.

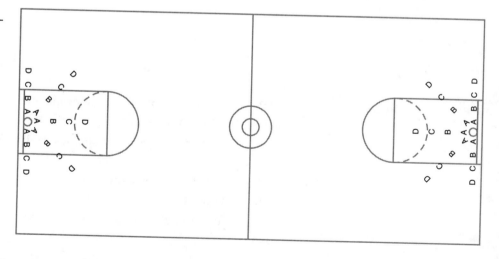

Notes	To make a game out of this, set a time limit. The winner is the player who completes the most angles in the allotted time.

Game Two

Name Around the World

Purpose To practice correct shooting form

Setup Divide the squad into two groups, one on each end of the court. Each player has a basketball. The shooting positions are shown in Figure 11.7.

Description A player shoots a layup from Position A. If he misses, he can "chance it" by taking a second shot. If he misses his chance, no matter what his shooting position is, he must return to Position A and begin over. If he makes either his first shot or his chance shot, he goes to the next position. If the shooter does not chance it, he begins his next turn at the position where he last attempted a shot.

FIGURE 11.7
Shooting positions for Around the World.

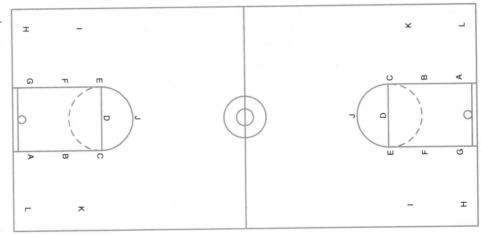

Notes
- Make a game out of this drill by allowing every player two starts; the player who advances the farthest wins.
- Use only Positions A–G for younger players. Use A–L for older players.
- Make it more difficult by requiring players to go around the world and back to where he began.
- Tailor the drill to reflect the skill and maturity level of your squad.

Rebounding Games

Following are two games to help your players work on their rebounding skills. The first game works on offensive rebounding, and the second one focuses on blocking out.

Game One

Name	Put-Backs
Purpose	To teach players to get an offensive rebound, pump fake, and score
Setup	Place two players around the basket and a coach at the free throw line (see Figure 11.8). If you have an assistant, you can have the same formation at the other end of the court.
Description	You shoot and intentionally miss the shot. The two players fight for the rebound. Whichever player gets the rebound is on offense; the other player is on defense. The offensive player attempts to score (he might need to pump fake to do so). If the defender deflects the ball outside the lane, you begin the sequence by shooting and missing again. Otherwise, the players keep getting the rebound and trying to score.

FIGURE 11.8
Setup for
Put-Backs.

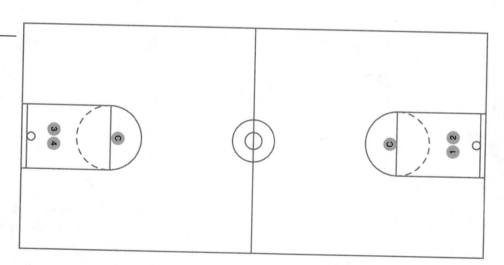

Notes	■ Make a game out of this by setting a two-minute limit and counting the baskets scored by each player.
	■ Combine this drill with Monkey in the Middle (described earlier in this chapter) to keep everyone active.
	■ To make the drill more difficult, use three players at a time instead of two.

Game Two

Name	Block Out
Purpose	To teach defensive players to block out and to teach offensive players to avoid block-outs
Setup	Play two-on-two under the boards. Place one offensive rebounder on the big block and the other offensive rebounder around the perimeter. You stand near the free throw line with the ball (see Figure 11.9).
Description	You shoot and intentionally miss your shot. On the shot, the defenders block out the attacker. The attackers try to avoid the block-outs and go for the offensive rebound. After 5 attempts, the rebounders on the block and the perimeter trade positions (but retain their roles on offense and defense). After 5 more attempts, the players switch offensive and defensive roles, and you repeat the 10 shots.

FIGURE 11.9

Setup for Block Out.

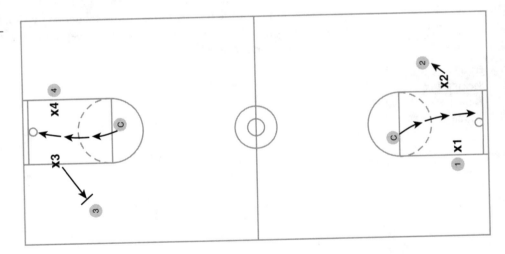

Notes	▪ Make the game more difficult by requiring the defenders to hold their block outs until the ball hits the floor.
	▪ Make a game out of the drill by counting the number of offensive rebounds followed by a score out of ten attempts. The offensive winner is the rebounder with the most scores. The defensive winner is the rebounder who allows the fewest scores without fouling.

Various Offensive Skill Games

In this section you'll find three games that work on different aspects of offense: footwork, passing and shooting, and posting up.

Game One

Name	Pivot Time
Purpose	To teach players with the ball to pivot to protect the ball without walking
Setup	Divide your squad into groups of 3 (see Figure 11.10). Place these groups of 3 at least 20 feet apart anywhere on the court. One of the players in each group has a ball. The other 2 players are defenders.
Description	The two defenders constantly try to grab the ball as the player with the ball pivots to protect it. After 30 seconds, the players rotate. A new player has the ball and the two other players try to steal it. After another 30 seconds, the third player in the group has the ball.

FIGURE 11.10

Setup for Pivot Time.

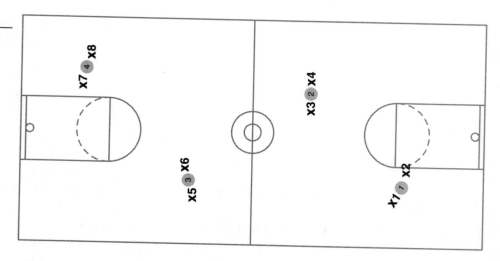

Notes	You can extend the time to one minute per player with the ball. But if you do this, allow the player to dribble two dribbles in any direction before picking up the ball. He may make this dribble anytime he feels he is in trouble. The other two players chase the ball, attempting to steal or deflect it.

Game Two

Name	Shoot n' Pass
Purpose	To teach players to shoot, follow the shot, rebound, and make an outlet pass
Setup	Place two players at each basket. One has the basketball (see Figure 11.11).
Description	The player with the ball shoots from the distance you want. She follows her shot. The player rebounds the made or missed shot. The player passes the ball to her teammate who has positioned herself at a spot on the floor prescribed by you (a good spot to receive an outlet pass). The player now goes to another spot on the floor while her teammate shoots, rebounds, and passes back out to the original shooter.

FIGURE 11.11

Setup and execution for Shoot n' Pass.

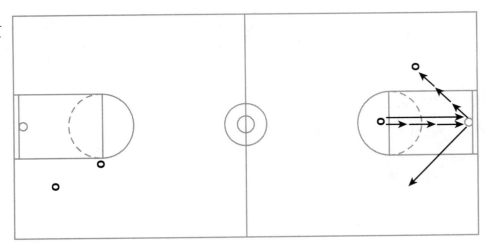

Notes	■ To make this a fun game, have the players at the opposite end of the court play a two-minute game against the players at the near end. The team that scores the most baskets wins.
	■ Combine this drill with Monkey in the Middle and have all players involved in one or the other drill at the same time.

Game Three

Name	Post Up
Purpose	To teach your players offensive moves around the post
Setup	Divide the squad into groups of three (see Figure 11.12). Place one player at the 45° angle on the arc on the left side and one at the

45° angle on the arc on the right side. Put the third player beneath the basket.

Description   The player underneath the basket breaks to the big block on the left side. He receives the pass from the player at the arc. The player performs the move you prescribe, rebounds his made or missed shot, and passes to the player on the arc on the right side.

This pattern continues until you say "Rotate." The three players rotate one position. Continue until all players have a chance to practice post moves.

FIGURE 11.12

Setup and execution for Post Up.

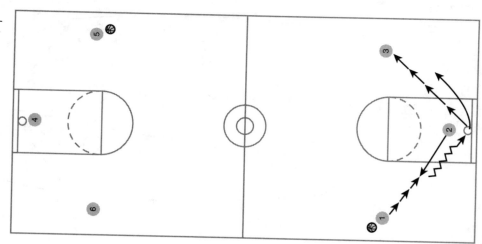

Notes   Younger or lesser-skilled players might only be able to perform the drop step from both sides of the basket. More highly skilled players might be able to perform the spin, the half-spin, and the up and under (a move in which the player fakes a shot and as the defender goes up to contest the shot, the attacker steps "under" for the layup, laying the ball under the arm of the defender).

Fast Break Games

The fast break is one of the more exciting plays in basketball. Here are a couple of games to help your players hone their fast break skills.

Game One

Name   Pass n' Go

Purpose   To teach players to rebound, outlet pass, fill the lanes, and finish the fast break with a score

Setup   Position two guards and three big men, in a two-three zone (or zone of your choice).

Description   You shoot and intentionally miss. A player rebounds and makes an outlet pass to a guard, and becomes the safety (see Figure 11.13). The guard passes to the other guard breaking into the middle lane. The four players fill the lanes

(your choice of players), with the fourth player becoming the trailer. The players finish the break with a score.

FIGURE 11.13

Execution of
Pass n' Go.

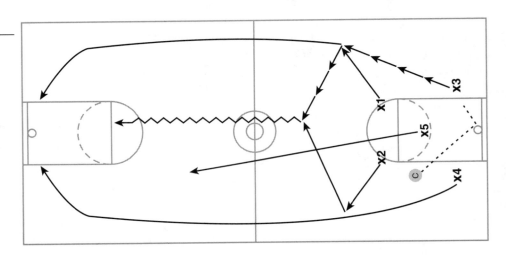

Notes   Adjust the fast break to your preferences. You can require the outlet pass receiver to dribble the ball to the middle lane instead of passing it there. Make adjustments according to your players' skills and maturity levels.

Game Two

Name   Three-on-Two Continuous Break

Purpose   To teach players to speed dribble, pass on the move, fill the three lanes of a fast break, and run a give-and-go offense

Setup   Divide the squad into three lines and place them at one end of the court (see Figure 11.14). Place two defenders at the other free throw lane.

Description   This is a two-part drill. In Part A, the three lines race down the floor in the three fast break lanes. These lines can be passing the ball or the middle lane player can be using the speed dribble. These three attack the two defenders at the other end of the court in a three-on-two fast break.

In Part B, the two defenders rebound the missed shot and attack the shooter (who is now the defender) in a two-on-one fast break to the original starting end of the court. The two nonshooters stay as the new defenders for the next wave of three-on-two attack. You can require these two new attackers to pass the ball instead of dribbling the ball. The defender tries to stop the attack by stealing or deflecting the pass.

FIGURE 11.14

Setup and execution for Three-on-Two Continuous Break.

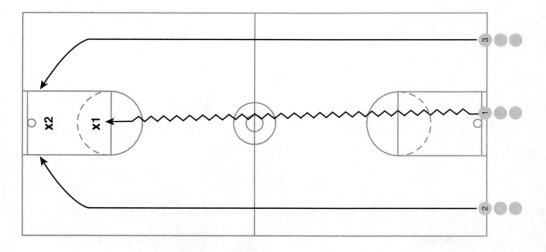

Notes

- Use only Part A if your players' skills or maturity levels hamper your use of both phases.

- Instead of attacking three on two, you can require the three players to use the give-and-go offense until they get a layup.

Special Plays Games

The following three games will help you prepare your players to work two of the oldest plays in the book—the give-and-go and the pick-and-roll—as well as an inbounds play.

Game One

Name	Give and Go
Purpose	To teach players to continuously give and go
Setup	Place six players on one end of the court, ready to go three-on-three (see Figure 11.15).

Description   This is a two-part drill. In Part A, use only the 3 attackers. These 3 players continuously pass and go. Two players execute the give-and-go. The third player fills a spot 15 feet from the original receiver. These 2 execute the give-and-go while the third player fills a spot for the next give-and-go.

In Part B, the three defenders are added and these defenders must jump to the ball on every pass and try to keep the give-and-go from being successful. No dribbling is allowed.

FIGURE 11.15
Setup and execution for Give and Go.

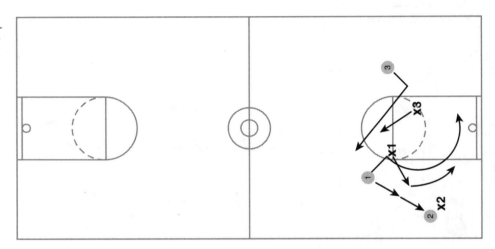

Notes
- Use only Part A if you wish to work only on offense.
- Make a game out of this by requiring the defense to stop the offense five times before the defense and offense switch duties (or before you bring new players into the game).
- Allow back door cuts, middle cuts (cuts through the middle of the lane), and screens as well, depending on what you want your players to work on.
- Use this drill to focus solely on your offense or to work both defense and offense at the same time.
- To win, count the number of possessions it takes before the defense has stopped the attack five times. The offensive winner is the team that scores the most before they are stopped five times. The defensive winner is the defensive team that allows the fewest baskets before stopping the offense five times.

Game Two

Name	Pick and Roll
Purpose	To teach the pick-and-roll
Setup	Divide your squad into two groups. Put two attackers and two defenders on
	each half of the court. Place any additional players as substitutes on each end of the court.
Description	An offensive player passes to the other and follows the pass with a screen on the defender on the ball (see Figure 11.16). The player with the ball dribbles around the screen and the screener rolls to the basket. The two defenders defend the screen as the offensive players execute the pick-and-roll.

FIGURE 11.16

Setup and execution for Pick and Roll.

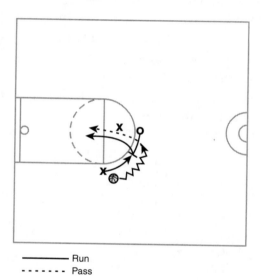

———— Run
- - - - - - Pass

Notes

▪ You can make this a two-part drill. In Part A, use only the offensive players. The two attackers run the pick-and-roll. After the players have learned the pick-and-roll, require the screener to roll to the basket and cut back outside for a pass. The passer then executes another screen and roll. This can be continuous.

▪ In Part B, add defenders. You can now make a game of it. Count the number of scores out of 10 attempts. The offensive winner is the group with the most scores; the defensive winner is the group with the fewest scores allowed.

▪ If your players have already learned the give-and-go (and the middle cut, the back door cut, and so forth), you can have them decide which offense to run. This keeps the defense guessing.

Game Three

Name   Inbounds Play

Purpose   To teach the team an inbounds play that works against both zone and player-to-player defenses

Setup   Divide the squad into two teams, one on each end of the court.

Description Player 3 takes the ball out of bounds (see Figure 11.17). On a set signal, such as slapping the hands on the ball, all players begin their movement:

■ Player 2 dips toward the middle of the court before breaking off Player 5's screen.

■ Player 2 cuts to the corner.

■ Player 1, who is the safety (the player who will receive the pass if no one else is open) breaks toward mid-court.

■ Player 4, meanwhile, comes over to screen for Player 5.

■ Player 5 comes off the screen and cuts to the basket on the weak side as Player 4 rolls to the basket on the strong side.

■ Player 3 inbounds to the player who gets open first, ideally one under or near the basket.

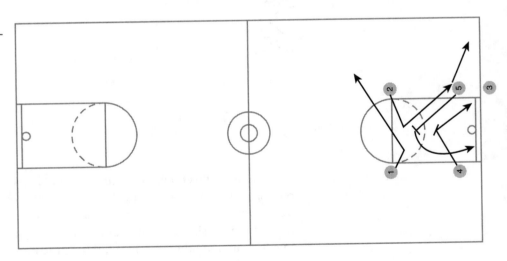

FIGURE 11.17
Setup and execution for Inbounds Play.

Notes   After your players have this play down, use a defense to defend against it. Try both player-to-player defense and zone defense. Run several possessions, and then switch the offense and defense around.

Individual Defensive Skill Games

Here are three games that focus on various aspects of individual defensive skills. They also play into team defense, but call more on individual effort. Following these three games, three more will be presented on team defense.

Game One

Name	Wave Drill
Purpose	To teach defenders all the steps and overplays needed to control the offensive player
Setup	Place all players on the court in a defensive stance in several lines (see Figure 11.18). You stand in front of them with a basketball in hand. All players must be able to see you.
Description	You begin with your left foot as your pivot foot. Do the steps of the Rocker Step. The defenders respond as if they are guarding you, using the appropriate foot movement (retreat step, advance step, swing step). Do this for awhile, and then dribble from a jab step. The defenders use the correct foot movement (the slide step). Go into as many dribbles as you feel you need. Then go back and start with your right foot as your pivot foot.

FIGURE 11.18
Setup for Wave Drill.

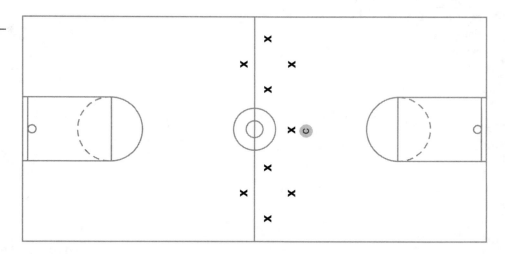

Notes	You can make this more difficult by making your movements quicker, requiring the defenders to read and react quicker.

Game Two

Name	Ball Side D
Purpose	To teach defenders to jump to the ball and deny the passing lanes
Setup	Divide the squad into groups of four. If it does not divide equally into sets of four, use one extra in each group and rotate. Two are on offense and two are on defense. Send one group to each end of the court (see Figure 11.19).
Description	Player 1 has the ball and is being harassed by X1. Player 1 cannot dribble to begin the game; he must pass to Player 2. X2 is in the passing lane between Players 1 and 2, trying to prevent Player 2 from receiving the pass.
	Players 1 and 2 pass back and forth as long as they can. After the initial pass, Players 1 and 2 can dribble to attack the basket. The defenders attempt to steal the ball, to deny good passes, and to deny baskets.
	Rotate the players from offense to defense. After several tries, rotate the players again: This time Players 1 and 2 switch, as do X1 and X2.

FIGURE 11.19

Setup and execution for Ball Side D.

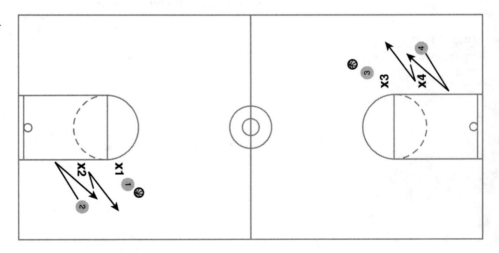

Notes	Award the defense a point for every tipped pass and two points for every steal. Take away a point from the defense for every pass completed in the lane or received in good shooting position.

Game Three

Name	Help Side D
Purpose	To teach defenders proper positioning on the help side, stop the breakaway dribbler, and defend the two-on-one break
Setup	Divide the squad into groups of three—an offensive player with the ball on one side of the court, a defender two-thirds of the distance between the ball and his assignment, and his assignment on the help side of the court (see Figure 11.20).
Description	This is a five-part drill. You can use any part separately, in combination with other parts, or as a complete five-part drill, depending on the skills and maturity of your players.

Part A deals with proper positioning. X2 should be one step off the line between the player with the ball and the defender's assignment. Player 1 should throw several passes in a line from herself to Player 2. X2, if she is in proper position, will deflect all these passes.

Part B deals with X2 "closing out" her assignment. Player 1 throws a lob pass crosscourt to get the ball to Player 2. X2 should be on Player 2 as the ball arrives. You can have Player 2 and X2 play one-on-one, or you can have Player 2 pivot into triple-threat position before passing the ball back to Player 1.

Part C deals with denying the flash pivot. Player 2 breaks toward the ball and X2 gets in the passing lane to deny the pass. Should the pass be completed, you can require them to play one-on-one, or you can have the Player 2 pivot into triple-threat position before passing back to the Player 1.

Part D has Player 1 driving to the basket. X2 comes off her assignment to stop the breakaway dribbler. You can require this to also be a one-on-one game.

Part E allows Players 1 and 2 to go two-on-one in a fast break situation against X2.

After X2 has been on defense through each of the parts, rotate the players until all have played all three positions.

Notes	If X2 deflects a pass or stops the offense, she gets a point. After all players have played all three positions, the defender with the highest point total wins.

FIGURE 11.20
Setup for Help
Side D.

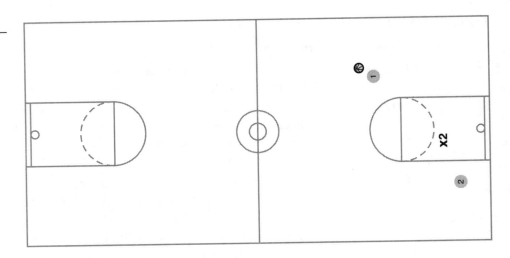

Team Defensive Skill Games

These final three games will test your players in their ability to play effective team defense.

Game One

Name	Shell Game
Purpose	To tie together all the defensive parts of the ball-side and help-side individual defensive drills
Setup	Play four-on-four. You will call out what you want the offense to do, or you can let them run any screens or cuts they wish.
Description	Player 1 has the ball and is covered by X1 (see Figure 11.21). X2 is on help side, so he is two-thirds the distance from the ball and Player 2 and is one step off the line between Players 1 and 2. X3 is also on help side, so he is two-thirds the distance from the ball and his assignment. X4 is on ball side, so he is denying the pass to Player 4.

From these positions, any of the parts in the Ball Side D or the Help Side D drills can be run, as well as the Give and Go or the Pick and Roll drills. For example, you can require the ball be passed around the perimeter and each defender has to adjust his positioning (two-thirds distance from ball to assignment and one step off the line with the ball). This means you are drilling only on proper positioning.

Or you could require the Help Side D drill be executed. In this case, Player 1 would try to pass the ball to Player 3. If successful, X3 would have to close out. The other defenders would have to adjust their positions. This is really a controlled half-court scrimmage without using post players.

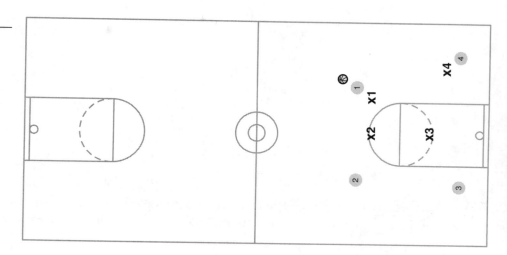

FIGURE 11.21
Setup for Shell Game.

Notes
- Give each group the ball 10 times. After 10 possessions, the team that scored the most baskets wins.
- Make the game more difficult by having the defense fast break after each possession by the offense. If the defense scores on the fast break, they get a point.

Game Two

Name	Screen Away
Purpose	To teach defenders to defend screens off the ball
Setup	Divide the squad into groups of three. Put three attackers and three defenders on each half court.
Description	This is a two-part drill. In Part A, the offense continuously runs screens away from the ball. In Part B, the defense defends against screens away from the ball.

Player 1 passes to Player 2 and goes to screen away on Player 3's defender, X3 (see Figure 11.22). If the screen away is not successful, Player 2 passes back out to Player 3, who reverses the ball to Player 1. Player 3 now goes to screen away on Player 2's defender, X2. This continues until you stop the action.

FIGURE 11.22
Setup and execution for Screen Away.

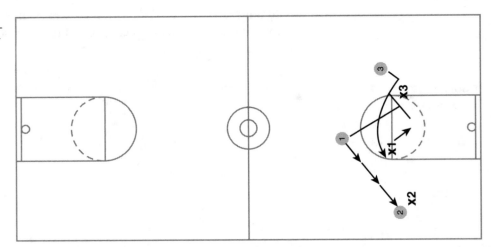

Notes

■ You can require certain passes by the offense. You can also make the drill more difficult for the defenders by allowing cutting as well as screening away.

■ You can make a game out of the drill by giving each team 10 possessions and counting the number of baskets each team scores. The defense gets a point for stopping the offense and the offense gets a point for scoring.

■ Rotate the offense and the defense and keep the count going. The winner is the team that scores the most points.

Game Three

Name   In the Zone

Purpose   To teach defenders their responsibilities and slides of the zone defense

Setup   Put five offensive players and three defenders on the court, as shown in Figure 11.23. The offensive player at the free throw line can move from side to side of the free throw line. The other offensive players remain stationary but are in a position to shoot as they receive the ball. The challenge is in three defenders stopping five offensive players from getting a shot off. You stand outside of the arc with a basketball.

Description   No dribbling is allowed in this game. You pass the ball to an offensive player who is open in the corner. The defense should begin by covering the high post player and the two players on the big blocks.

The defender on that side of the court rushes out to cover the corner. The high post defender drops to cover the big block. The opposite defender on the big block moves slightly toward the basket.

The corner player with the ball can now either pass to the high post or back out to you. If the pass goes to the high post, the defender on the big block races out to cover the high post. The defender in the corner races to cover the just-vacated low block.

This passing continues until there is a breakdown in the zone defense and the offense has a good shot to take. Three defenders should be able to prevent a shot from the five attackers if the attackers are not allowed to move or dribble.

FIGURE 11.23
Setup for In the Zone.

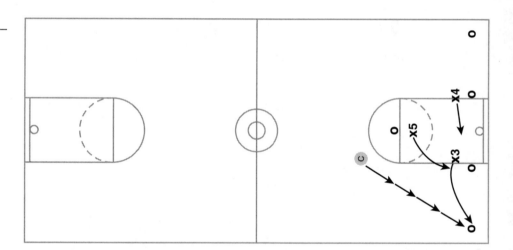

Notes

Give the defense a point for every pass they deflect, two points for every steal, and subtract a point for every shot the offense takes and two points for every basket they make. The major purpose of the drill is to prevent shots by hustling in your zone defense. After 10 possessions, rotate 3 other defenders onto the court. The 3 defenders that score the highest win the game.

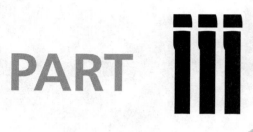

PART III

APPENDIXES

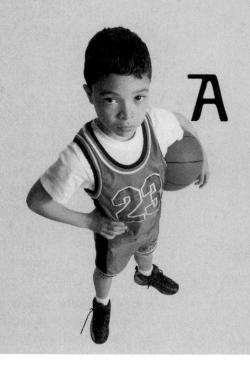

SAMPLE LETTER TO PARENTS

Note: This is a sample letter to parents of 6- and 7-year-olds. Your message to parents of older players would likely be a little different. Adjust the letter according to your needs, regardless of the age of your players.

Dear Parent(s):

I'm excited about the new season approaching, and I know you and your child are, too. I want to take a moment to introduce myself and let you know my approach to coaching.

I've been coaching for three years in the park district, beginning when my oldest son entered the league, and am certified in first aid/CPR. Over the years, I've developed this coaching philosophy:

- The child is more important than winning. We will do our best to win, but helping each child develop his or her skills, learn more about basketball, and enjoy the experience—while providing for everyone's safety and well-being—take precedence over winning.
- Everyone gets equal playing time.
- We practice using games and drills that simulate what the players will experience in real games. We do this to practice skills and learn the rules of the game.
- I use positive reinforcement and plenty of encouragement as kids learn the skills. Basketball is a tough sport to master. My focus is to help players learn the fundamental skills and understand the basic rules and strategies of the sport.

What do I expect from the players? I expect them to show up to practice on time, to respect and listen to me, to respect their teammates, to try their hardest, and to have fun. I structure practices so the learning is fun.

What do I expect from parents? I expect them to

- Get their child to practices and games on time or to let me know if they're not coming
- Encourage and support their child and the team during games
- Refrain from booing or making negative remarks to the referees or the other team
- Get involved in a variety of ways with the team (I'll fill you in at the first practice on these opportunities)
- Practice, if at all possible, with their child at home (I'll give you ideas for what to practice)

Please understand that basketball has some inherent risks. Injuries can occur—generally minor, such as scrapes or bruises. I will do everything possible to run an injury-free practice, and I do know how to respond in case of an injury, but I do want you to know the chance of injury always exists in basketball, as in any other sport.

Our first practice is Monday, December 12, 5:30 p.m., at Blair Gym. At that practice I will give you a full practice and game schedule. I will also give you a medical information sheet to fill out; this will let me know whether your child has any special medical conditions and who to contact in case of an emergency.

I'm eager for the season to start! See you on December 12.

In the meantime, feel free to contact me at 342-3537 before the first practice, or at any time during the season. Thanks for your attention to this letter, and I look forward to a great season coaching your child!

Sincerely,

[Name, phone number, address]

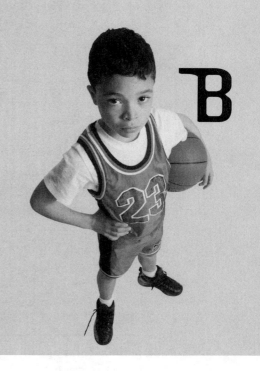

MEDICAL EMERGENCY FORM

Child's name _____ D.O.B. _____ Date _____

Address _____ Phone _____

IMPORTANT INFORMATION:

1. Does your child take daily medication? Yes ___ No ___

If yes, please explain:

_____

_____

_____

2. Does your child have any drug, food, or insect allergies? Yes ___ No ___

If yes, please explain:

_____

_____

_____

3. Does your child suffer from ___ asthma, ___ diabetes, or ___ epilepsy?
Check all that apply.

4. Will your child be bringing any medication to practices or games? Yes ___ No ___

If yes, please name the medication and explain its purpose:

_____

_____

_____

5. Has your child had a tetanus shot? Yes ___ No ___

6. Is there anything else pertinent regarding your child's health or physical condition? Is yes, please explain:

_____

_____

_____

List two people to contact in case of an emergency:

Parent or guardian's name _____ Home phone _____

Address _____ Work phone _____

Second person's name _____ Home phone _____

Address _____ Work phone _____

Relationship to child _____

Family doctor _____ Phone _____

Family dentist _____ Phone _____

Health plan name _____

Health plan ID# _____

Parent or guardian's signature _____

Date _____

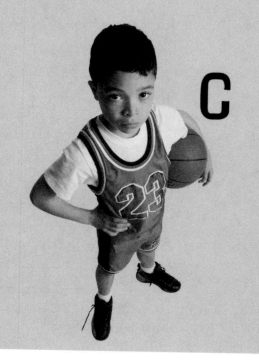

C

INJURY REPORT

Name of child _____

Date _____

Time _____

Description of injury:

_____

_____

_____

_____

_____

_____

First aid administered:

_____

_____

_____

_____

_____

_____

Additional treatment administered:

_____

_____

_____

Referred to:

_____

_____

Signature of person administering first aid:

_____

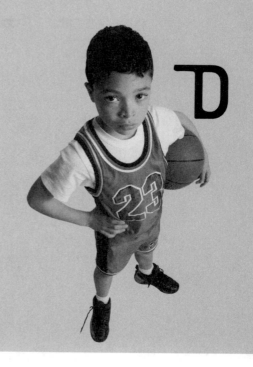

SEASON PLAN

Week	Purpose	Tactics/Skills	Rules
1			
2			
3			
4			
5			
6			
7			
8			

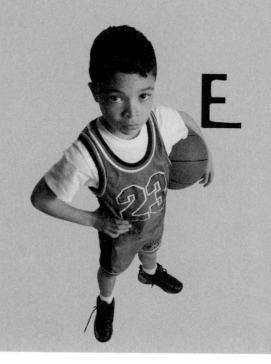

E

PRACTICE PLAN

Date _____ Place _____ Time _____

Equipment _____

Purpose _____

Activity	Description	Time	Comments
1. Warm-up			
2. Activity 1			
3. Activity 2			

Activity	Description	Time	Comments
4. Activity 3			
5. Wrap-up			

Notes:

_____

_____

_____

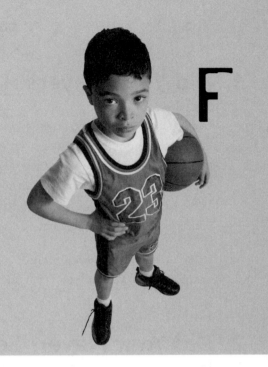

F

SEASON EVALUATION FORM

Note: Fill this out at season's end. Rate yourself honestly and use this form to note your areas of coaching excellence and areas for improvement for next season. Also consider giving a copy of this form to a couple of outside but interested observers who could give you an objective evaluation (in other words, not your spouse or your best friend!).

There are 14 main areas to consider. Respond to each statement, scoring yourself between 1 and 5, based on this scale:

1 = very poor

2 = poor

3 = average

4 = good

5 = very good

Note that similar statements will appear in more than one area; this is because the issue affects multiple areas.

1. Did Your Players Have Fun?

Statement	Rating: 1–5
The practice and playing environments were positive and enjoyable.	
I effectively organized practices.	
My players learned the skills they needed to be competitive.	
My players experienced individual successes in practices and games.	
I doled out playing time appropriately.	
I reinforced players' competence and helped them see positive aspects of their performance.	
I didn't overemphasize winning.	
Overall, I would say my players had fun playing basketball this season.	

2. Did Your Players Learn New Skills and Improve on Previously Learned Skills?

Statement	Rating: 1–5
My ability to teach skills enabled my players to learn what they needed to learn.	
I pushed player development of skills at an appropriate rate, neither too fast nor too slow.	
I helped all my players improve and didn't just focus on a certain set of players.	
I adjusted my teaching plan as necessary, according to the skill levels of my players.	
I planned and conducted practices effectively.	
I encouraged and supported my players as they continued their growth.	
Overall, I would say my players learned new skills and improved on any previously learned skills they had.	

3. Did You Help Your Players Understand the Game and Its Rules?

Statement	Rating: 1–5
I presented game-like situations for players in practice so they could gain a better understanding of how to respond to similar situations in games.	
I taught my players the appropriate rules and strategies of the game.	
My players showed, through their play, that they understood the basic rules and strategies.	
Overall, I would say I helped my players understand the rules and strategies of basketball.	

4. Did You Communicate Appropriately and Effectively?

Statement	Rating: 1–5
I let parents know my coaching philosophy before the season began.	
I let players and parents know what they could expect from me and what I expected from them.	
I communicated clearly with players, parents, referees, other coaches, and league administrators.	
I kept parents informed and maintained a healthy flow of communication with them throughout the season.	
My players understood my skill instruction.	
My communications with my players were positive and authoritative.	
I was well-prepared for delivering the technical instruction my players needed.	
My players were prepared to respond appropriately in various game situations because I had prepared them for what they would encounter.	
My players paid attention to me when I spoke.	
My body language was in sync with my verbal messages.	
I was a good listener and focused on reading my players' body language and hearing and responding to their comments and questions.	
Overall, I would say I communicated appropriately and effectively with everyone involved.	

5. Did You Provide for Your Players' Safety?

Statement	Rating: 1–5
I was trained in CPR and first aid.	
I warned my players and their parents of the inherent risks of basketball.	
I had a well-stocked first aid kit on hand at practices and games and was prepared to use it.	
I knew of any allergies or other medical conditions of my players and how to respond regarding those conditions.	
I checked the practice and game courts for safety hazards and eliminated those hazards, if possible, before playing on the courts.	
I enforced rules regarding player behavior that enhanced player safety.	
I provided proper supervision throughout each practice.	
I offered proper skill instruction so players were prepared to play the positions I put them in.	
I took water breaks as appropriate during practice.	
Overall, I would say I adequately provided for my players' safety.	

6. Did You Plan and Conduct Effective Practices?

Statement	Rating: 1–5
Players paid attention to me because I had a purpose to what I was doing.	
There was no down time in practice while I was trying to figure out what to do next.	
Players were active and engaged at multiple stations that I ran simultaneously; they weren't standing around waiting for a turn.	
I used games and drills that were designed to teach a specific skill or tactic I wanted my players to work on that day.	
My players learned new skills and refined ones they already had.	
My players had fun in practice.	
I had fun, too.	
Overall, I would say I adequately planned and conducted effective practices.	

7. Did Your Players Give Maximum Effort in Practices and Games?

Statement	Rating: 1–5
I didn't yell at players for mistakes and for their general quality of play.	
I didn't compare one player to another.	
I didn't create long lines in which players had to wait their turn.	
I taught players the skills they needed to know.	
I gave players specific technique goals to work toward.	
I provided specific, positive feedback.	
I encouraged my players, especially when they got down, and praised correct technique and effort.	
I genuinely cared for my players and let them know I cared about them and their achievements.	
I helped players take home the positives of the practice or game.	
I praised hustle, desire, and teamwork shown in practices and games.	
I ran efficient, purposeful practices in which players were active and engaged the whole time.	
I valued each child for his or her own abilities and personality.	
I didn't play favorites with my players.	
I listened to my players.	
Overall, I would say my players gave maximum effort in practices and games.	

8. Did Your Players Leave the Games at the Gym?

Statement	Rating: 1–5
I coached my players to keep the game in perspective—to give it their all but to let it go if they lost, and to not get a big head if they won.	
My players were not too high after a victory. They came back prepared to practice and play.	
My players were not too low after a loss. They came back prepared to practice and play.	
I talked appropriately with any of my players who were either too high or too low after a game, helping them to leave the game at the gym.	
I talked appropriately with any player who had difficulty mastering his emotions at the gym or immediately after a game. I steered the player toward mastering his emotions.	
I helped my players focus on the next game, regardless of the outcome.	
Overall, I would say my players left the games at the gym.	

9. Did *You* Leave the Games at the Gym?

Statement	Rating: 1–5
I didn't make too much out of a victory. I came back prepared to coach.	
I didn't get too low after a loss. I came back prepared to coach.	
I kept control of my emotions, win or lose.	
Overall, I would say I left the games at the gym.	

10. Did You Conduct Yourself Appropriately?

Statement	Rating: 1–5
I communicated in positive ways with opposing coaches and players and with referees.	
I coached within the rules and had my players play within them.	
I maintained control of my emotions in practices and games while providing the coaching and support my players needed.	
I kept the games in perspective and helped my players do the same.	
If I ever lost my cool, I admitted my mistake and apologized for it.	
I was an appropriate role model for my players.	
Overall, I would say I conducted myself appropriately as a coach.	

11. Did You Communicate Effectively with Parents and Involve Them in Positive Ways?

Statement	Rating: 1–5
I had few or no misunderstandings with parents regarding my coaching philosophy.	
I delegated responsibilities, sharing the workload with many parents and making my program stronger in the process.	
I wasn't as stressed as I might have been, had I not involved parents.	
I appropriately addressed the few misunderstandings or concerns parents had.	
Overall, I would say I communicated effectively with parents and involved them in positive ways.	

12. Did You Coach Appropriately During Games?

Statement	Rating: 1–5
I kept my strategy simple and based it on my players' strengths and abilities.	
I helped my players get mentally prepared for a game by focusing them on the fundamentals they needed to execute and on the game plan.	
I provided tactical direction and guidance throughout the game.	
I was encouraging and supportive.	
I gave technique tips and reminders and let the kids play, saving the error correction for the next practice.	
I tended to the kids' needs during the game—emotional and psychological as well as mental and physical.	
I helped players keep the game in proper perspective.	
I used a positive coaching approach.	
I effectively rotated players in and out.	
My players conducted themselves well during and after the game, including the post-game handshake.	
I held a brief post-game meeting, giving the kids some positives to take home, regardless of the outcome of the game.	
Overall, I would say I coached appropriately during games.	

13. Did You Win with Class and Lose with Dignity?

Statement	Rating: 1–5
I and my players shook hands with the other team, offering them congratulations.	
I thanked the referees for volunteering their time.	
My team celebrated victories fully and in a way that showed respect for the other team.	
My players didn't hang their heads after a loss, no matter how hard the loss was.	
I helped the players regroup and take home positives from games we lost.	
Overall, I would say we won with class and lost with dignity.	

14. Did You Make the Experience Positive, Meaningful, and Fun for Your Players?

Statement	Rating: 1–5
My players still had the same zest and enthusiasm at the end of the season that they did at the beginning.	
My players seemed to want to come back for another season.	
My players learned the skills, tactics, and rules of the game.	
My players learned about themselves, learned what it means to be a member of a team, and grew up a bit.	
Overall, I would say the experience for my players was positive, meaningful, and fun.	

Index

How can we make this index more useful? Email us at indexes@quepublishing.com

How can we make this index more useful? Email us at indexes@quepublishing.com

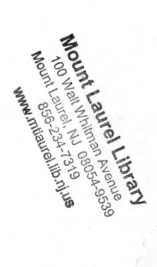